"As I was savoring every word, I kept thinking how I wish I had this wh[...] wonder, if someone had helped me dig deep into my own curiosities back t[...] more fully? This is a brilliant guide, and a lovely opportunity to explore wh[...] to choreograph a life, and a death, on your terms."

—**Gabrielle Elise Jimenez**, hospice nurse; end-of-life doula; conscious dying educator; and author of four books: *Soft Landing*, *The Hospice Heart*, *At the Bedside*, and *What Would Gabby Say?*

"This compassionate preparation guide is a valuable resource for anyone looking to deepen their understanding of how to prepare and plan for the end of their life. Francesca provides a wealth of information on the practical and emotional aspects of end-of-life planning—including exercises that prompt self-reflection and wishes for the future—that guides readers on a journey of self-discovery."

—**Jennifer Mallmes, BGS**, facilitator and developer of the End-of-Life Doula Program at Douglas College in Canada, and cofounder of the End-of-Life Doula Association of Canada

"*The Death Doula's Guide to Living Fully and Dying Prepared* by Francesca Arnoldy provides readers with the tools to incorporate a healthy awareness of death as they navigate life. The practical reflections and exercises included in the book can calm fears of death and catalyze growth in consciousness and joy. This workbook should be on every kitchen table to bring essential conversations about mortality back into day-to-day life."

—**Karen Wyatt, MD**, retired hospice physician, host of *End-of-Life University Podcast*, and author of *7 Lessons for Living from the Dying*

"A thoughtful, kind, compassionate, forgiving, loving, and infinitely practical lesson in living well and dying your way. No surprise it comes from the desk of an end-of-life doula."

—**Jessica Zitter, MD, MPH, FAAHPM, FCCP**, author of *Extreme Measures*, and founder of Reel Medicine Media

"Whether facing your own death or caring for someone at the end of theirs, this remarkable book can become a true friend and guide on the journey. With care and wisdom, Francesca has crafted a comprehensive workbook that tackles the practical and spiritual dimension of dying. In it we explore our fear, make meaning of our life, heal the past, and sort out end-of-life wishes. A tall order beautifully executed."

> —**Johanna J. Lunn**, founder of the When You Die Project, and award-winning filmmaker whose work includes *Saying Goodbye* and *Architecture of Death*

"A beautiful portrait of the human capacity for love, acceptance, and meaning as we face life's end. Rich in deep experience and thoughtful reflection, *The Death Doula's Guide to Living Fully and Dying Prepared* is an emotionally wise book that provides the framework for people in any life stage to engage in death journaling and death wellness. Francesca gently and compassionately guides us on a journey that will inspire you to reflect on your own life and help you to be meaningfully present for those nearing the end of their lives."

> —**Christopher Kerr, MD, PhD**, hospice physician, researcher, and author of *Death is But a Dream*

"*The Death Doula's Guide to Living Fully and Dying Prepared* blends insights, tools, and resources from Arnoldy's years of experience as an end-of-life doula into a workbook for building a healthy relationship with life and death. It is a gift for all readers: inspiring us to contemplate how we want to live today and the positive impact we hope to leave behind, and helps people facing death find clarity and closure in their final days, weeks, or months."

> —**Kim Callinan**, president and CEO of Compassion & Choices, the largest end-of-life care consumer advocacy organization in the US; and certified death doula

"This is a well-organized, generous encouragement toward death wellness, grounded in compassionate action. Accessible exercises and practical resources for doulas, care partners, and curious people exploring their relationship with mortality."

> —**Dina Stander**, end-of-life navigator, burial shroud maker, and founder of the Northeast Death Care Collaborative

The Death Doula's Guide to

Living Fully
and
Dying Prepared

An Essential Workbook to Help You Reflect Back,
Plan Ahead, *and* Find Peace on Your Journey

FRANCESCA LYNN ARNOLDY

New Harbinger Publications, Inc.

Publisher's Note

This publication is designed to provide accurate and authoritative information in regard to the subject matter covered. It is sold with the understanding that the publisher is not engaged in rendering psychological, financial, legal, or other professional services. If expert assistance or counseling is needed, the services of a competent professional should be sought.

Any personal stories from the author are recounted solely from perspective and memory. Names and identifying details of clients have been changed to protect privacy.

The pronoun "they" will be used as plural as well as singular for gender inclusivity

NEW HARBINGER PUBLICATIONS is a registered trademark of New Harbinger Publications, Inc.

New Harbinger Publications is an employee-owned company.

Copyright © 2023 by Francesca Lynn Arnoldy
        Reveal Press
        An imprint of New Harbinger Publications, Inc.
        5674 Shattuck Avenue
        Oakland, CA 94609
        www.newharbinger.com

All Rights Reserved

Cover design by Sara Christian
Acquired by Ryan Buresh
Edited by Gretel Hakanson

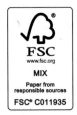

FSC
www.fsc.org
MIX
Paper from
responsible sources
FSC® C011935

Library of Congress Cataloging-in-Publication Data

Names: Arnoldy, Francesca Lynn, author.
Title: The death doula's guide to living fully and dying prepared : an essential workbook to help you reflect back, plan ahead, and find peace on your journey / Francesca Lynn Arnoldy.
Description: Oakland, CA : Reveal Press, an imprint of New Harbinger Publications, Inc., 2023. | Includes bibliographical references.
Identifiers: LCCN 2023000799 | ISBN 9781648481369 (trade paperback)
Subjects: LCSH: Death. | Grief. | Terminal care.
Classification: LCC BF789.D4 A72 2023 | DDC 155.937--dc23/eng/20230310
LC record available at https://lccn.loc.gov/2023000799

Printed in the United States of America

25   24   23

10   9   8   7   6   5   4   3   2   1   First Printing

I dedicate this book to my many teachers, especially my client "C,"
who taught me how to connect with people on *their* terms as well
as the lesson that we all live and die in our own way.

And my humble thanks to you, dear readers. I'm certainly not the first
person to write about death, and I won't be the last. I didn't invent the idea
of preparing for the end. I am but one of many who recognize the
importance of developing a healthy relationship with our mortality.

Contents

Part I: Orientation: Developing a Foundation of Compassion

Part II: Preparedness: Opening to Death Wellness

Part III: Pause and Practice: Strengthening Your Coping Techniques

Foreword

I first met Francesca Lynn Arnoldy in my role as a developmental psychologist/human development specialist teaching in the Human Development and Family Science program (HDFS, formerly Family Studies) at the University of Vermont (UVM). Francesca was a student at UVM from 1999–2003, and she graduated as an HDFS major. Through our program, Francesca studied two central lenses through which to consider individual development—lenses that are evident in her approach to doula work and especially in how she interacts with readers throughout the pages of *The Death Doula's Guide to Living Fully and Dying Prepared*.

The first lens is the Life Course Framework; this calls our attention to the interaction of historical events, early life experiences, and individual decisions and opportunities in affecting later life outcomes (for example, Elder and Shanahan 2006). The second lens is Bronfenbrenner's Ecological Model of Human Development (originally articulated in his 1979 book). This model focuses our attention on how various environmental contexts affect our development while also considering how individuals themselves impact their environmental contexts. A core concept in this model is that of ecological transitions. As Bronfenbrenner (1979) described these, such transitions occur when "a person's position in the ecological environment is altered as a result of a change in role, setting, or both" (26) and "every ecological transition is both a consequence and an instigator of developmental processes" (27). Professor Lawrence Shelton (2019, 53), another of Francesca's professors in HDFS, explains "ecological transitions provide the person opportunities or challenges to adapt to the new setting or role."

As I read this book, I saw evidence of both these lenses. Francesca treats death, the dying process, and preparing for both (as the person who is dying and as those who must prepare for life without a loved one) as developmental opportunities. She recognizes that facing our mortality is essentially an ecological transition that presents us with new opportunities and challenges, and that is affected by our life course to date. Through her book, Francesca offers us, her readers, an array of activities and reflections, along with her caring and comforting presence that shines through the pages, to support our preparation for this final transition.

End-of-life preparation may take place following a terminal diagnosis, but the book is designed for all of us as living beings to anticipate and plan for our own and our loved ones' dying and death. In fact, many of these activities may be easier to approach when not directly confronting a serious illness. I am experiencing this firsthand with a good friend who recently received a terminal diagnosis. As she self-isolates and puts much energy into not thinking about dying and death, I find myself wishing that she had this book just a few months ago, and that she and I had worked through many of the activities together, sharing our hopes and fears around life's end. Those conversations could serve to hold her and her loved ones now, even as she focuses her energy away from the reality of her diagnosis. Of course, I would expect her perspectives on dying to continuously evolve, but the earlier conversations and activities could have served as groundwork from which to build, both for my friend and for we who love her.

At the core of this new publication, Francesca offers us, her readers, a map that is both broad and intricate, with multiple pathways we might take to better understand ourselves and engage with the final phase of life. That she supplies a map is not surprising as it is a common thread throughout her body of work. First, in *Cultivating the Doula Heart: Essentials of Contemplative Care* (2018), Francesca offers would-be doulas a map for how to understand and become a caring and compassionate doula. In her second book, *Map of Memory Lane* (2021), Francesca's beautifully written and illustrated children's book, she offers another kind of map—a memory map—for young children to imagine before a loved one's death, and for them to follow after a loved one's death. This picture book also offers adults a way to open up a conversation with children about mortality and help them imagine loss while also helping them understand that love remains within our memories.

Now, through this third book, Francesca offers a guiding map to help readers approach our own final developmental transition—from living to dying, from life to death, and from living relationship to memory. Simultaneously, the workbook provides a map for how to be present for and support our loved ones' preparation for this final transition. What readers will also find by working through this book is that it is sure to facilitate gentle introspection and a deeper engagement with life itself. The irony of this book, focused as it is on death, is that it really offers a means to living more fully, through to its end.

—Jacqueline S. Weinstock, PhD
The University of Vermont

Introduction

Welcome.

I am so pleased you've found your way here. And I feel honored to provide you with a guided tour through the profound work ahead, which is essentially what I offer to people as their doula. Broadly described, doulas support others through times of intensity—labor, birth, illness, death, or grief—with boundless compassion and steady courage.

Since 2009, I have assisted countless clients, friends, loved ones, and neighbors to plan for and experience these unparalleled life transitions. Through workshops, presentations, and training programs, I have taught thousands of people key doula philosophies and practices, the best of which are infused into these pages. Basically, I have emptied the contents of my "doula bag" into this workbook—my most-trusted techniques, approaches, and activities.

When offering to support people, I first present an array of offerings and then encourage them to decide what resonates. Please keep this in mind as you begin your efforts. Don't feel pressure to complete each and every prompt and exercise included. Instead, in accordance with your goals and current bandwidth, always feel invited to:

- peruse and choose

- try and modify.

You might start with the chapters that feel most important and then jump around from there. Or you might take many months to slowly work through each page in order, deciding to engage in activities or not as you go. No matter your particular path, make sure to enjoy a sense of completion and fulfillment along the way.

What to Expect

The overarching aim of this workbook is to supply helpful guidance for examining your inner workings, creating remembrance gifts, and preparing for your last chapter—whatever your current health status.

Discovery of self → Sharing of self → Making plans

The book is highly interactive and includes a wide variety of thought-provoking prompts. There are seven steps involved, each with a distinct purpose.

Part 1 (Orientation): Develop a foundation of compassion.

Part 2 (Preparedness): Open to death wellness.

Part 3 (Pause and Practice): Strengthen your coping techniques.

Part 4 (Processing): Explore what feels unfinished and undiscovered.

Part 5 (Projects): Clarify and share your authentic self.

Part 6 (Planning): Draft your wishes for care.

Part 7 (Parting Gifts): Say goodbye.

The topics and trajectory of these sections stem from my many years supporting people through birth and death—life's epic thresholds. As an educator and doula, I prioritize customized, empowering care for every person I have the honor to serve. Each client experience deepens my reverence and affirms the benefits of healthy preparedness for these most significant periods. When people have not had important conversations ahead of time, others are left to guess, which adds stress to phases already rife with complexity.

You might still have some questions and even fears at this point. *Who is this book for? What exactly will I learn and do in this book? What qualifies this author to be my guide through it? What will mortality work entail?* Let's go through some answers together.

Who Is This Book For?

This workbook is for anyone willing to lean into these layered subjects, including but not exclusively:

- adults ready to begin or revisit plans for their eventual death

- people with a serious or terminal condition looking to prepare for their final phase

- people practicing conscious living who want to explore conscious aging and dying

- honorary or biological parents, grandparents, aunts, and uncles, as well as godparents, guideparents, mentors, or guardians who want to create remembrance gifts for those they care about

- people hoping to lessen their fear of death

- deathcare workers, family or volunteer caregivers, and professional care providers supporting others through the end of life.

Some readers will begin contemplating mortality and documenting their life, death, and care wishes while their health is stable, perhaps sparked by a notable transition, loss, or another type of awakening. Others might feel motivated due to illness or the aging process. As your guide through this process, I aim to inspire you to acknowledge—and even reclaim—what it means to be mortal because I have experienced the benefits of these efforts personally, and I have witnessed positive outcomes for others.

I became a deathcare worker by way of birth. Initially, as a birth worker, I focused on the postpartum period, helping families adjust to life at home with a new baby. Then, I became a childbirth educator and, a few years later, a birth doula (meaning a nonmedical care person who provides informational, emotional, spiritual, and physical support before, during, and after childbirth). Over the years, my mind opened to the endless constellation of possibilities during labor and delivery, and so did my heart. I found that my work untangled and exposed hidden assumptions about what was *best* for my clients. And so, I softened into a stance of curiosity as opposed to righteousness, releasing any strict agenda of how things "should" go during this great transition.

After a handful of years as a birth doula, my family endured a number of losses within a short span. Two of my grandfathers, my father-in-law, and our dog died. Each death was different, and they all offered profound lessons as part of their legacy. I noticed myself naturally shifting into my doula presence during those heart-rending times.

What we were going through seemed so unpredictable, yet I felt the need to nurture trust in the face of all that felt unknown. I found myself slowing down and proceeding with heightened senses. I paid attention to how others were acting and reacting and tended to their diverse needs. I found myself leaning into the mysterious nature of dying while studying the experiences keenly. The organic translation of my birth-doula presence to the dying period not only seemed to calm and comfort others, but it also inspired me to explore how to hold space at both bookends of life.

In terms of my personal mortality awareness, it wasn't until I became a parent that it really occurred to me how impactful my dying would be on those I love. Parenting younglings coupled with myriad losses, big and small, compelled me to begin my *death journal*—what I've named my remembrance scrapbook. Truth be told, I cannot recall which entry was the first one, as it has been many years in the making, and I freely skip around its pages. Likely, it was a written message—words too weighty to hold inside any longer. Then, a few more notes (all dated) followed by some special poems, song lyrics, articles, quotes, mantras, lists, and mementos.

Now, my death journal sits at the ready for when it is needed. My closest family members know of its existence and purpose. I have also included information about my end-of-life care preferences. Every now and then, I add to it, filling up the blank spaces with encouraging refrains and comforting sentiments.

My death journal allows me to prepare, in advance, reassurance and guidance to those who will miss me most. Selfishly, I hope it will also allow me to surrender into my time of dying with slightly less resistance, as I suspect worries about family will be my heaviest anchor to this lifetime. I anticipate feeling more ease knowing I have created a gift like no other—a treasure most mourners yearn for following a significant loss. And by writing this workbook, I aim to bring some of that ease to you and yours as well.

How to Work with This Book

This book contains many activities as well as ample space for writing. Some readers will utilize it as a draft of sorts—a place to jot down ideas as they surface. Then, they will compose final versions to store or share. Others will work within these pages, and the entries will suffice as complete. Either approach or a hybrid of both is entirely acceptable. Customization is highly encouraged! You can download worksheets and activities from the website for this book, http://www.newharbinger.com/51369.

Although this book is organized with scaffolding to build upon as we progress, this is your path. You can choose what to complete and when to complete it. If you decide a section does not apply or appeal, bypass it. You might return to it, you might not—your call. Conversely, if you find yourself meandering down an unexpected side trail, see where it goes. You might very well find additional ways to expand beyond these pages.

Death journaling requires substantial courage. It asks you to acknowledge your impermanence, which is no small task. This is human work though, and each of us is naturally capable of it. Plus, the potential rewards of these efforts are infinite, including feeling lighter and liberated to live life more fully.

Still, some people will have doubts upon beginning this journey and might ask some of the following questions.

Will it be depressing? Depressing? Generally not—at least not overwhelmingly so. Poignant? Yes. Profound? Often. It is reasonable to expect moments of heartache and even regret while reminiscing on the life you have lived, those you have loved, and saying goodbye to it all. Still, contemplating death tends to be a gratifying practice. It opens our eyes. We wake up! We realize our time is limited. We pay closer attention to what is happening and develop a deeper appreciation for each good day, knowing it is one less in our grand tally.

Mortality awareness immerses us into the present moment. The only way we can act upon the past is by processing and healing from it. The only way we can affect the future is by setting intentions and making mindful decisions. When we're able to see things in this way, we understand the current moment is brimming with potential.

Death wellness practices enable us to release some of the heaviness we carry. When we live aware of our mortality, we can regularly take stock, consider what needs mending, and act upon it. By uncovering fears and verbalizing hopes, we lift emotional burdens. And we consider our legacies—all we've done and all we leave behind. We find comfort in the creation of meaningful gifts and messages for our dear ones. We find solace in knowing there will be fewer disagreements between family members before, during, and after our time of dying, because we have spelled out wishes in advance.

What if my loved one(s) dies before me? For the most part, we cannot know the length of our life or that of others. Death journaling will help reveal what feels unresolved so you can spend time now repairing relationships, if that feels necessary, or strengthening them, and addressing what may have gone unsaid. I encourage you to speak the words you hold in your heart while you still can and also write them down for later. Both are powerful actions.

What if I do not have someone to receive my writing? Not everyone intends to share their journaling, and sharing isn't necessary. If you don't have someone to receive this book once you've completed it, and this distresses you, try to navigate those feelings as adaptively as you can. Perhaps a recipient will emerge while doing this work. Or that might not happen. Still, it won't negate the value of your efforts.

Death journaling is part of an ongoing practice of processing, planning, and preparing that will continue throughout your remaining days. Even on its own, introspection is just as worthwhile as the development of remembrance gifts for others. People have different goals and circumstances. All are valued here.

Will thinking or talking about death make it happen? Some people worry that contemplating mortality will bring death closer or cause it to happen sooner. This type of fear can often be dispelled by thinking about the many providers and educators who have dedicated their careers to deathcare and who have done this work for decades. Yet, all fears are valid and deserving of thoughtful consideration. If you have this type of worry and it is rooted in a cultural, religious, or spiritual tradition you grew up within (or some other equally influential source), please know there is no need to defend or explain it. Something—a need or desire—has brought you to this workbook. Follow your heart and create your best way forward.

What if I am very ill or facing imminent death? First, please feel the care and concern I wrap around your shoulders. What a complex time. I will not attempt to guess at the many challenges you are facing, as this is your unique path and your interpretation of it is what matters. But I assume your attention is being pulled in many directions.

Make sure to honor your energy levels without setting unreachable goals. You will balance spending time being present in the moment with taking time to reflect on the past, alongside any other concerns that may be on your mind. Perhaps there is someone in your care circle who might assist you with this workbook so you can preserve some of your strength for other efforts. May the activities you are able to complete here offer you a sense of accomplishment and peace.

To Each Their Own Lens

We each carry our own goals and agenda into our death awareness work. As a human being, you are a bountiful collection of genes and characteristics, and you're also shaped by foundational and transformative moments. Your individual lens, which you view the world through, informs how you integrate information; factors including your race, ethnicity, age cohort, country of origin, culture, belief system, family environment, identity, lived experiences, and past conditioning influence your outlook. As you move through the chapters of this book, gently note what aspects of your personhood you would like to celebrate, restore, or perhaps shift to be in alignment.

Ultimately, many of the prompts and exercises ahead focus on the creative exploration of your mortality, values, legacy, and wishes for care. While the process is quite encompassing of life and death matters, here is a list of what your workbook is *not*.

A repository for secrets. When surviving family members open my death journal, it will not reveal hidden details. They will not discover a whole new side of me. They will find me—familiar me—as they knew and loved me. By drafting entries, I am creating a place for loved ones to visit my essence and the memories we shared.

A quick fix for a broken heart or for the fear of death. Some readers will arrive at the beginning of this book laden with grief following a major loss, while others might be harboring intense existential anxiety. Some carry both. There is no fast track through either. There are no easy, universal answers. We cannot bypass the time and energy necessary for integration and healing if we aim to be healthy and whole. The only way through struggle is to work through the thick of it, and the process differs from person to person. Death journaling can be a significant part of resolution though, as it includes thoughtful reflection and honest expression.

A medical or legal document. There are helpful worksheets in the appendices that are precursors for advance care planning, and the work you do within this book—for instance, in articulating your wishes for care at the end of your life—will likely inform some of the information you can include in formal records. But this book is not intended to be a medical or legal document. Many countries (and regions within countries) have specific templates available that enable you to specify your legal and medical preferences as well as to elect a decision-making surrogate for times you might not be able to verbalize your wishes. Do some research to explore your local options, getting assistance as needed from caregivers and family, and talk with your primary care provider and a legal professional for more details.

Potential Hurdles

As you are starting this workbook, you might have reservations or expectations. It's important to be prepared for possible challenges that can keep you from making progress.

Writer's block. Some people feel apprehension about writing. This is common. Sometimes this comes from doubting our aptitude. *Am I skilled enough to write well?* Please know, this workbook is not a research paper or formal dissertation. It is *you* on a page. When shared, it is a generous act of kindness and love. Spelling errors, grammatical slips, and pen smudges help keep it real, and realness is what people tend to crave when dealing with loss.

Sometimes fear of writing comes from a deeper place. You might question, "How will this be received?" And you might wonder what your loved ones—and generations to come—will think of what you've written. Ultimately, death journaling is a process of illuminating essentials. By expressing inner thoughts, we become vulnerable. First, we uncover our authenticity, and then we find the courage to convey it. Go slowly and build trust in yourself as you do this work.

The perfect moment. Perfect moments are elusive. If we wait for conditions to be *just so* to create our death journals, they will likely remain empty. Excuses and distractions are readily available, and this work is intense. My personal motivational mantra to prevent procrastination is: *You'll never have more time than RIGHT NOW.* Another trusty one I use is: *Sit and start.* What might be yours?

_____

_____

Conversely, it is not advisable to force yourself to complete this entire book in a day. You will need to take breaks to allow thoughts to percolate. I often make better sense of things while walking through the woods, for instance, or pulling weeds in my garden. So, when you find yourself wrestling with a question, try to get fresh air or find some other way to relax and open to insight.

Ultimately, in mortality work as with everything, balance is key. My hope is you will find this journey emotionally rewarding, and momentum will build upon itself. You will feel inspired and intrigued, and thus drawn to your writing perch.

Internal messaging. When we engage in introspective activities, our inner voice can sometimes be judgmental and harsh. We might doubt we've lived a life of worth or that we have interesting stories to share. We might question our value. Sometimes we feel guilty for "burdening" others when expressing our woes or requesting support, fearing they're wasting their time and energy on us. We tend to be harder on ourselves than on anyone else.

Clinical psychologist and author, Lisa Firestone (2013) describes this critical inner voice as an "internal enemy, which is hidden among your more objective and realistic views and reactions." We often experience it as a running commentary that attacks and criticizes our actions and interactions in everyday life. It can generate shame and embarrassment while undercutting confidence, holding us back from actualizing our plans and becoming our most authentic selves. Here are some tips for managing your internal messaging when needed.

- Question the validity of the messaging. Consider it objectively. Imagine a friend in the place of yourself. What would you say to your friend in that case?

- Question the root of the messaging. Whose standards, expectations, or rules are associated with it? Are they in alignment with your current attitudes about yourself and the world?

- Place the messaging in a speech bubble in your mind and trust it will pass by like clouds in the sky. Remind yourself that everyone struggles with this issue sometimes. It is part of being human.

While journeying through mortality work, you'll want to make sure the voice that resounds above all others is one that is true and purposeful. With intention and practice, you can start to notice and quiet any unkind mental monologues that occur. And in response, you can nudge yourself forward with encouragement and patience.

Working in Community

Consider death journaling with others if it is appealing and possible—either with loved ones or with support from a therapist, doula, or hospice worker. As author and teacher Rachel Naomi Remen (2001, 338) once put it, "After all these years I have begun to wonder if the secret of living well is not in having all the answers but in pursuing unanswerable questions in good company." If you choose to work through this book with friends or family members, note that each participant will find their most ideal method of engagement. Make allowances for variety, as it will enhance everyone's experience.

Working in partnership will not spare you the trek into the recesses of your individuality. Instead, you will journey in parallel, with each of you retreating inward to complete whatever work you're being asked to do and then reemerging to debrief together. After all, this arrangement is not unlike the dying process in the sense that kind companionship can be immensely reassuring, and yet, in the end, we must each travel into death as a solo voyager.

Whatever your plan for this workbook might be at this point, let's dive into our first journaling prompt. Here are some steps you can follow.

1. Find an available spot that is cozy and free from clutter so your body can be comfortable and your mind can focus.

2. Take a few slow deep breaths and set aside any worries, knowing you can return to your regular mode after you finish.

3. Read the following prompt, and then allow your thoughts to flow freely as you record them by hand. Your writing can be neat or messy. You can write in complete sentences or scribble notes. There is no right or wrong way. You are finding *your* way.

What brought you to this mortality work? What goals or intentions do you hold as you enter into these practices?

_____

_____

_____

_____

_____

_____

_____

_____

Reflections

Read over your entry. Were you able to write freely? Did you find yourself trying to direct your words or make logical sense of them? Were any of the goals or intentions you documented surprising or unanticipated?

Take a moment to congratulate yourself for beginning! Expect moments ahead of uncertainty as you both question and fortify your points of view. Anticipate an array of tears, laughter, frustration, and a deepening sense of contentment as you unearth what makes you, you.

Before continuing, choose one prominent goal from your writing that stands out and enter it below as your "bold intention" to reinforce its strength.

My bold intention: _____

May it be so.

Final Tips for the Work Ahead

The activities to come will summon your full attention and openness. You will spend time exploring your inner realm and assessing coping techniques—both the ones you've established and some you might wish to cultivate. You will recall sources of happiness and comfort as well as wistful moments. You will review "quality of life" considerations while determining what "quality of death" means to you. Throughout your contemplation, remember:

1. Meet yourself where you are and discover where you'd like to go…and ultimately end up.

2. Keep sources of motivation and sustenance handy to combat procrastination because, as the saying goes, "It often feels too early until it's too late."

Letter to Care Partners: Using This Guidebook as a Supportive Tool

"As you grow older, you will discover that you have two hands, one for helping yourself, the other for helping others."

—Sam Levenson, actor, humorist, and bestselling author
(O'Toole 2013)

First, please know, you are held in gratitude. Whether you are a clinician, faith leader, deathcare worker, life coach, volunteer, neighbor, or loved one, the support you supply to others is crucial. Without it, many among us would feel lonely and neglected. So, thank you.

Many readers will be guiding themselves through this workbook. Some will, instead, turn to a trusted person like yourself for help with this task as it might feel too overwhelming to complete alone. Or they'll want your companionship through a process they anticipate will bring ease and peace. As someone who cares for others, you are invited to utilize this text as a tool for assisting clients, patients, workshop participants, friends, or family members with their death awareness practices and end-of-life preparations. An imperative preliminary step, though, is to do your own mortality awareness work first. Otherwise, as care providers, we simply cannot hold the hands of others with adequate authenticity through challenging conversations or periods.

When we're unclear about our personal preferences, we risk operating from a place of clouded judgment, and we might even project our ideal course of action onto someone else. This can cause harm because we'd be quieting the other person's voice versus lifting it up. We might also take on someone else's anxieties as our own if we're not mindful, which can be incredibly draining. We have to be able to differentiate what is *ours* from what is not. In other words, we need to come to terms with our own impermanence and consider our specific wishes first, so we can clearly delineate our thoughts, feelings, and preferences from those belonging to our loved ones, clients, or patients.

A special note for those who are supporting people facing the end-stages of a condition: Even though you are also mortal, it is imperative to understand that a terminal disease brings people into a different headspace. While you might have strong feelings about certain care decisions, they are largely theoretical, while the other person's experience is unfolding in the present moment with much more urgency. Please keep this distinction in the background of your mind.

Getting clear on our own preferences is not our sole prerequisite as carers, though. Hospice nurse, doula, and author, Gabrielle Elise Jimenez (2022) affirms, "To provide care for people who are dying, and for those who are grieving, we must be at peace with ourselves. We cannot walk alongside someone else when we are riddled with our own grief, pain (physical or emotional), stress, or exhaustion." Working through this book will likely uncover unhealed wounds and help you access the resources—internal and external—needed to support yourself and others through times of intensity, like the end of life.

Professional Care Providers

Throughout the process of grappling with mortality, many questions will arise. Due to your role, those you serve will look to you for suggestions—and even answers. Your patients or clients will seek your counsel regarding sensitive topics.

Likely, you will have related information to share due to your knowledge of research and interventions in addition to your past work experiences. You are an expert in your field, which is undoubtedly beneficial, yet your patients or clients know themselves best. You must meld all sources of wisdom together to offer truly person-centered—ideally, person-led—care.

Instead of providing solutions, you can frame suggestions as options. Empower each patient or client to actively participate in discussing choices. Communicate not only the possible benefits and risks of an option, but also realistic expectations, and then ask the person you're working with how it all sounds. Ask how well the options align with who they are and what they want. As a provider, you can collaborate with those receiving your care to create customized approaches that honor every person's uniqueness.

Making Suggestions and Sharing Stories

Making time for discussions as well as quiet listening are key approaches to compassionate care. Is it also appropriate for care providers to make suggestions or share stories? Yes—judiciously and with caution. It's best to first allow someone time to talk without interruption. They might be able to come to their own conclusions. If additional information is warranted, how can you dispense it while promoting each patient's or client's sense of agency?

Before speaking, pause, WAIT (ask, "Why am I talking?"), and ponder:

- Who is this share benefiting? Do I want a turn in the spotlight? Do I want to sound wise? Am I trying to fix or rescue this person?

- Am I attached to the outcome—to their decision? Am I pressuring my patient or client? Might they feel worried about disappointing me?

As a doula, when I feel compelled to share an example that is potentially helpful, I try do so in an anonymous, general way. If the story is from my personal life, I usually do not pose it as such. Instead, I might begin, "I know of someone who considered/benefited from..." or "I worked with someone who..."

There are several advantages to this approach. First, by removing identifiers, I convey to my clients I will carry their experience forward with respect as I am demonstrating my commitment to confidentiality. Second, a neutral example leaves more room for clients to objectively consider the situation. It's a more open, inviting approach.

In general, patients and clients appreciate:

- being seen as their true self

- being heard and having their input genuinely considered

- being treated as a partner in their own care

- having time to discuss next steps at any juncture.

Friends or Family Caregivers

As a friend or family member (chosen or biological), you might be supporting a dear one who has chosen to begin this workbook. Or, you might have picked up this book because you're interested in having someone you care about try it—and you may not be sure if they'll agree.

Ultimately, whatever your particular situation, you can decide to either (1) move through these exercises in advance of guiding your person through them or (2) complete them with your loved one side by side. You are both human. You are equals. You do not need to be an expert on all things related to life's end. Instead, you can make time for important conversations, assist your person with brainstorming questions to ask during their appointments, and do your best to stay present and supportive as you work through exercises simultaneously.

What if time is short, but your person does not show interest in mortality awareness practices? It is never our place to pressure or guilt someone into doing this work. We can be invitational though, which empowers individuals to maintain self-determination. This is hugely important as a serious illness tends to render someone increasingly dependent. People often feel quite powerless against the force of a terminal diagnosis. Sensitivity to this effect is paramount.

How, then, can we be invitational? Perhaps by focusing on ourselves first. This workbook is for any adult at any point. Instead of inquiring about your friend or family member's preferences, ask to discuss your own fears and wishes; for example, "I know talking about advance care planning isn't easy, but I've been thinking about my own preparations lately, and I'd like to share them with you if that's okay." If the person is agreeable, it can open further communication or at least get them thinking about matters related to their care.

Tips for Supporting Others Through Death Wellness Work for Any Care Partner

Although your specific reasons for utilizing this workbook as a care tool are unique, here are some overarching tips to encourage positive experiences.

Get as clear as you can on your own planning. Formulating your own preparations for life's end will help you clarify priorities and enable you to create ample space for someone else's process. The activities within this book, coupled with formal advance care planning documents, cover a comprehensive array of information you can record for yourself and also share with others.

Continually revise your end-of-life forms. With time, your relationships and perspectives will change. Regularly assess what you have written to ensure it is up-to-date. You might commit to revisiting forms on your half-birthday, on New Year's Day, or on National Healthcare Decisions Day (United States) every April 16.

Respect each person's distinct pacing. When faced with an intense, pressing reality, we tend to lean into it at certain moments and turn away at others. This is a built-in, protective mechanism that fosters emotional health. Be mindful of particular points when the person you care for might be willing to lean in or might need to turn away. Forcing someone to accept what feels overwhelming about their situation can damage their well-being and any trust you've built. Care for others with patience and compassion.

In terms of compassion, let's define what it is and discuss how it differs from the two other tools you might use as a caregiver: sympathy and empathy.

Sympathy vs. Empathy vs. Compassion

As approaches to support, both sympathy and empathy have the potential to deplete a caregiver. Compassion, however, is mutually generative in terms of energy and meaning. This is the orientation we strive for when engaging in work with those contemplating the end of life. Semantics can be subjective, of course, and there is gray area between each of the three terms. The goal of differentiating them is to hone a modality that enables you to sustain your passion for your work.

Here are some definitions of sympathy, empathy, and compassion for you to consider (adapted from my 2018 book *Cultivating the Doula Heart: Essentials of Compassionate Care*):

What is sympathy? "I feel sad/bad for you." Sympathizing means feeling sorry for someone. It involves conjuring up an emotional state of pity in response to someone else's state of difficulty. When we sympathize, we take on a feeling that was not originally ours. We attempt to connect and demonstrate understanding by sharing in sorrow. We commiserate, yet by doing so, we chance compounding challenging situations by adding in our own heavy emotion.

What is empathy? "I feel how this feels for you." Empathizing means attempting to envision how we would feel in the other person's situation or remembering how we have felt in a similar circumstance. By overlaying our imagined experience onto their reality or our past onto their present, we believe we are meeting someone where they are. This responsive feeling can never exactly match the emotions of another person though, as this is not possible. Emotions are fluid and personal.

Sympathy and empathy, while well-intentioned approaches to offering solace, can become exhausting. Instead of being fully available and attentive as a supportive presence, we can end up expending energy feeling sad for someone or attempting to feel what they are enduring. Trying to match our emotional landscape to that of another can deplete our energy.

What is Compassion? "I honor how this feels for you." Compassion moves beyond empathy. It means learning how someone feels by becoming an ally and witness to their experience. When we practice compassion, we transition from the Golden Rule ("Do unto others as you would have them do unto you") to the Platinum Rule (coined by Dr. Milton Bennett in the 1970s): "Do unto others as they would have done unto them."

We make no assumptions. We allow others their reactions by remaining steady and centered while conveying our acceptance. We give people adequate space to navigate their best path. We encourage a thoughtful slowing down when those in our care might otherwise feel rushed to reach *the other side* of a challenging episode. We nurture courage as people confront chaos.

At the same time, we recognize our shared humanity in the common condition of suffering. As a fellow human, we know pain. We know hardship. What we do not claim to know is how another person views and manages their own hardship. When we create room between what is *ours* and what is *theirs*, we find this separation leads to more genuine connection because our understanding is not based on an effort to harbor shared misery.

Compassionate caregivers do not dip into internal reserves to refill another person's emptiness. Instead, we believe in the intactness of each person and their limitless potential to evolve and heal. We stay close and cultivate trust in each person's inherent wisdom and strength. We know that people are entitled to the completeness of their journeys as well as access to adequate support. Through our regard for innate wholeness, people are invited to see it for themselves.

As author and activist Parker Palmer (2016) once said, "The human soul doesn't want to be advised or fixed or saved. It simply wants to be witnessed—to be seen, heard, and companioned exactly as it is. When we make that kind of deep bow to the soul of a suffering person, our respect reinforces the soul's healing resources, the only resources that can help the sufferer make it through."

Practicing compassion as such revitalizes us. We can care for others without emptying ourselves. We feel honored that others invite us into their tender times of vulnerability. I encourage you to bring this compassionate spirit to those you serve and to offer this same kindness readily to yourself as well.

From my heart to yours,

Francesca

Self-Preparation: Heart Centering

While you work through entries, you will be inhabiting a particular head and heart space. It is beneficial to intentionally shift into an open, centered state as a preliminary step. If you already have an established technique for this, please continue with it. If you would like to explore other options, here is one to try and modify.

After you become familiar with the script by reviewing it a few times, you can guide yourself through it silently. Alternatively, you can record yourself reading the script aloud and listen to the recording. Make sure to speak slowly and leave pauses throughout so you do not feel rushed. The wording does not need to be exact. Use phrases that appeal to you.

Finally, note this exercise focuses on the breath, so it may not be appropriate or effective for those experiencing breathlessness. There are alternative options that utilize other senses or capacities listed after the script. (This exercise is inspired by Healing Touch therapy.)

First

Find a spot that is comfy and inviting. Ease yourself into your seat or bed and relax your muscles as much as you can, scanning yourself for tension from head to toe. Find as much comfort as possible in and around your body. Choose to gently close your eyes or hold a soft gaze.

The Script

Begin to slow your breathing, feeling the air coming in through your nose and out through your mouth. As you draw in your breath, picture a word that stands for pure well-being. Any word that comes to mind is the right one for you. Try not to judge the word that appears. Simply allow and welcome it.

Breathe that word in through your nose, and then send it down into your heart space. With each inhalation, feel it entering your heart and filling it up. Watch as your word grows and expands throughout your heart space from top to bottom, front to back, and side to side.

Breathe and fill. Breathe and expand.

Once your heart space is completely saturated with your word, begin to also breathe it outward on your exhale. Send it throughout your whole body, top to bottom, front to back, and side to side.

Breathe and send. Breathe and expand, taking as much time as you need to reach your whole body.

Once your entire body is saturated with your word, begin to share it beyond yourself and into the space surrounding you. Breathe it outward.

Breathe and send. Breathe and share.

Now pause and enjoy this full immersion into the abundance of well-being you have created. This space is yours. This is a space of healing.

When you're ready, begin to bring yourself back to the present moment by wiggling your toes and fingers. Remember, you can retain this sense of calm and return to heart centering whenever you like.

Reflections

Take a few moments to reflect on this practice. How was it for you?

_____

_____

Visualizations can be incredibly powerful, yet they are not right for everyone. If this exercise didn't resonate, please don't interpret it as a failure of sorts. Right now, you are in the process of reviewing strategies to determine which ones you will lean on and which you will sidestep. You're getting to know yourself and your preferences.

How might you alter this practice to best meet your needs? And how can you deepen it?

_____

_____

_____

Alternatives

Here are some other ways you can reflect on the word you've chosen to represent what "well-being" means to you.

Explore your word artistically (figuratively or literally). Gather art supplies of your choosing or from what is readily available. You might sketch with a pencil, paint with acrylics, collage with magazine cutouts, or sculpt with clay. Your word can become a color or symbol. Just as young children do not question their creativity, practice allowing and welcoming yours to come through.

Freewrite about your word. On a fresh piece of paper or within a blank file on a computer, begin to write any thoughts that come to mind about your word. Quiet your logical mind that grasps for order. Instead, allow and welcome revelations.

Explore your word musically. If you play an instrument, start a jam session with your word in mind. What sounds or melodies arise? Are they new, or do you find yourself playing a familiar tune? If you sing, begin by humming and vocalizing your word. Does a rhythm develop? Again, allow and welcome the process.

Take your word on a movement meditation. However and wherever you are able to move, take your word with you. Hold it in your thoughts. Perhaps repeat the word in unison with your movements. Then, allow and welcome your thoughts to expand around the word.

Final Thoughts

Once you find what works well for you, keep it available. Whether it is guided imagery, an artistic visual you can display, a meaningful sentiment you can repeat, or a song, utilize this practice as preparation for the sections to come. Your chosen go-to technique can help calm your nerves and allow insights to emerge with more ease as you engage in death wellness exercises.

Part I

Orientation: Developing a Foundation of Compassion

The goal of this section is to orient yourself in terms of presence and mindset. Your North Star, the value that will guide you in this work, will be compassion by way of connection. As the meditation teacher Sharon Salzberg (2015) puts it, compassion "challenges our assumptions, our sense of self-limitation, worthlessness, of not having a place in the world, our feelings of loneliness and estrangement. These are narrow, constrictive states of mind. As we develop compassion, our hearts open."

As you engage in mortality awareness practices, you will act as your own doula. Originally, "doula" was an ancient Greek title for women who assisted child-bearing women. It has roots in servitude and even slavery, but since the latter part of the twentieth century, there has been an effort to reappropriate the term. At present, "doula" is defined as a nonmedical care provider who offers emotional, physical, informational, and spiritual support to people going through major life transitions, such as birth and death.

When I begin working with clients as their death doula, I first explain the scope of my role and potential services to see what appeals. In turn, my clients identify their initial goals and interests. From there, the process follows a distinct trajectory:

Exploration of their personhood → Sharing of themselves → Preparing and planning

Your work in this book will follow this same trajectory. We'll explore your present and past, likes and dislikes, greatest achievements, and biggest heartbreaks. The investigation will always be invitational, never forceful. You're free to respond in as much or as little detail as you choose. These efforts will help illuminate your authentic identity, to yourself, in ways we don't often get to do in regular life.

From there, you'll start to map out how you might share yourself, your stories, and any messages you'd like to leave for your loved ones. This naturally transitions into more formal planning as you consider end-of-life care options. Ultimately, it's only once we have uncovered our inner workings that we can begin to envision how to honor them.

As mentioned, throughout the forthcoming activities, you will lean on yourself just as my clients lean on me as their doula. Even if and when there are other caregivers and providers available, it is still vital for a person to act as their own ally and advocate. In the end, you are your most enduring support system, and this book doles out the tools needed to become such.

CHAPTER 1

The Doula Way

For doulas to be present for others or themselves during monumental transitions requires the cultivation of a particular embodied approach. The qualities of this approach can be remembered by using the word DOULA:

D – Dedication to presence

O – Open-mindedness

U – Understanding with compassion

L – Listening intently

A – Allaying distress

In this chapter, we'll explore these techniques in order to build a solid basis for death journaling and mortality work. Let's go through each step of DOULA to clarify these interrelated components.

Dedication to Presence

While supporting others through times of intensity, doulas practice the art of holding space by creating a safe atmosphere where people can feel and express any kind of emotion while working through issues with honesty. As your own doula, you will hold space for your practice by cultivating an internal environment that feels spacious and welcoming.

When you pause, center, slow down, and shift into a healing presence for yourself, you become a container for the complex work of mortality exploration—just as you did in the opening "Heart

Centering" exercise. You make yourself a site for potential existential struggle and euphoric discoveries. Creating this space requires you to take an active role in self-preparation; holding that space asks you to *be* more than *do*.

In moments when you need to rededicate yourself to mindful presence or any of the DOULA qualities, using a mantra might be useful.

One that works well for presence is: *Vessel of calm, well of trust.*

How can you improve the quality of your healing presence? First, think of a time you experienced the healing presence of someone else. This could be a dear friend, family member, teacher, therapist, or any kind-hearted person who offered you concern and attention during a difficult episode. Sit in silence for a few moments to contemplate the following prompts, and then write your response by hand.

Think of a time you received sincere support from someone who genuinely cared. Describe the interaction and note what the person offered that felt so remarkable.

_____

_____

_____

_____

_____

_____

_____

_____

_____

Reflections

How was it to recall this interaction? Was it uplifting to revisit? It may have brought up memories of a tough period, which can be unsettling. If so, take this opportunity to implement some of the beneficial techniques you noted in your writing. What can you give yourself right now that the person supporting you offered back then? Take time for nurturance and then return when ready.

When I ask people to describe the presence of those who have supported them, they often use terms like *steady*, *quiet*, or *accepting*. When they explain how the person made them feel, they recall feeling seen, heard, and validated. Do these concepts mirror your experience? Are there other descriptors that were more or less prominent? How might you carry forward and emulate the care you received in the ways you treat yourself?

_____

_____

_____

_____

Open-Mindedness

The key to being open-minded as your own doula is curiosity. When we remain open to learning, we continually broaden our awareness. If instead, we enter into mortality work thinking we know exactly who we are and what we want, we limit our growth potential.

Societal or familial norms might leave you feeling pressured to view the end of life in a certain way. However, you might not yet be aware of all the options or perspectives worth considering. In such moments, the common phrase "You don't know what you don't know" rings especially true. We know what we have been taught, told, and shown, but dealing with death means dealing with the supreme enigma. You now have the opportunity to liberate yourself from imposed constructs. Try to remain malleable and intrigued by what surfaces, from reassurance to resistance and everything in between.

> Mindful mantra: *Uncertainty can inspire fear or curiosity—my response is my choice.*

Become your own *emotional ally* by committing to being a kind companion to yourself no matter the twists and turns ahead. Mortality work will change you if you let it. You will uncover amazing facets of your personhood.

Practice: Wonderment

Over the next day or two, find opportunities to integrate awe—a practice that brings the qualities of *presence* and *open-mindedness* together. Let your attention linger over the brilliance of a flowering house plant or the rhythmic swaying of a tree. Cue yourself to see life through fresh eyes, from the mundane to the extraordinary. No matter the subject of your focus, soak in the details and invite wonder.

Write about your practice here if you'd like.

_____

_____

_____

_____

Understand with Compassion

Doulas tune in to the discomfort found in liminal space—the space between one phase and the next—knowing it is through the struggle of hardship that we find the resolve needed to endure and, ultimately, discover our truest sense of self. Doulas also know that even when shattered by despair, people are fundamentally whole and intact.

As you contemplate mortality, you will likely feel some waves of anguish. You will want to turn away from what hurts. Please remember in those tender moments, your wounds are fertile ground for healing—not in the sense of a quick fix or cure, but in the sense of an unbroken soul, no matter what the body and mind endure.

Mindful mantra: *My whole self serves me—my scars and my strength.*

This does not mean you should forcefully expose any trauma you have faced, nor rush into the darkest parts of the journey before you feel ready. Compassion requires patience and sensitivity to yourself and your own capacity in each moment.

Lean in, and then take a breather. When you're ready, lean in again. Find your best tempo. Remember: You are entitled to the completeness of your experience, and you have the reserves and wisdom required. You are the antidote to distress; you are the source of catharsis.

Listening Intently

A core element of the doula role is listening. Doulas utilize silence while inviting someone to recount a memory, relationship, or their life in general. Gifting someone focused time to create a narrative can facilitate their acceptance of what has happened and can even foster meaning-making. With intention, doulas take care not to condone or condemn, while ensuring those receiving care don't feel alone or abandoned in their time of need.

This unfaltering openness is what you will be supplying to yourself. This book will act as your story-catcher. These pages offer quiet receptivity as well as reliable availability, always awaiting your willingness.

Mindful mantra: *My truth is legitimate. My words are testimony.*

Please know, your thoughts are valid. You have the right to your doubts and assertions. As you are completing exercises, try not to let input from others (either in real-time or from the past) derail your process when it doesn't feel valid. Also, continuously quiet the chatter in your mind that can interrupt your flow—especially that critical voice that attempts to minimize your confidence. Discern the messaging, rooted in fear, which holds you back from finding yourself.

When it becomes challenging to hush the noise that blocks insight, you might benefit from taking a break. Shift your focus for a period, knowing you can return to your work later when you have more energy. During your reprieve, you might:

Move your body. Even subtle movements while in bed or a chair can help when feeling stuck. Shrugging your shoulders or clenching a muscle group (for example, making fists or pointing your toes) and then releasing the tension might feel beneficial. In part 3 of the book, we'll review relaxation techniques you might also find useful.

Enjoy nature. If it is possible and appealing, go outside for your break. If it isn't possible, consider bringing the outdoors inside in the form of a flower, leaf, or handful of snow.

Try freewriting. Simply put pen to paper, writing anything that comes to mind with no agenda. Purge your mind until it feels lighter. Sometimes, when we stop trying so hard to make sense of something, insights can appear more freely.

Allaying Distress

Doulas aim to avoid escalating challenging situations or dynamics by making a conscious effort not to be swept along in the emotional current of others. It's a type of anchored composure that naturally encourages others to slow down and settle inside themselves as well. While engaging in mortality work, embody the practice of anchored composure to bring calm and comfort to yourself.

> Mindful mantra: *I have all I need, in and around me.*

While death journaling, you might feel overwhelmed at times. Older losses will likely wash over you. Notions tied to the stark concept of nonexistence might flood you. Give yourself permission to feel what you need to feel and even wallow in darkness for a period when that seems necessary. Then, allow yourself respite from the heaviness as you recenter your focus. Witness your efforts with kind eyes and a warm heart.

Tips for Strengthening Your Doula Presence

As you continue to harness the DOULA qualities over the course of your mortality awareness work, there are certain techniques that can bolster your efforts, enhancing your ability to be a steady, present, compassionate guide to yourself. They are as follows:

- Minimize distractions.

- Remain observant.

- Invite harmony.

- Value yourself.

Minimize distractions. As you complete the exercises in this workbook, prepare by first adjusting your surroundings. Our minds are easily stimulated. Competing demands, addictive devices, or even birdsong can break our concentration. It is not easy to maintain targeted awareness for substantial periods of time. Turning off a noisy radio or television and notifications on your computer can decrease distracting temptations.

Remain observant. When you feel yourself tuning out, let that be a cue to refocus your attention. You might even whisper a quiet reminder: *Tune back in.* Our minds will wander, yet we can gently redirect, again and again, in order to strengthen our ability to sustain focus for longer stretches. Also, recognize when you need to take breaks.

As another way to practice being observant, you can activate the part of your mind that notices patterns, synchronicities, and opportunities for contemplation even outside of this workbook. As you continue with the exercises, you will likely find connections between your past and present, between your wounds and anxieties, as well as between your lived experiences and expectations. Notice any themes that arise, which might hint at conditioned beliefs. Softly ask: *Do they serve me well?*

Invite harmony. During introspection, you needn't constrain yourself with preset boundaries. Instead of viewing death awareness practices through a lens of polar opposition (an idea must either mean *this* or *that*), acknowledge a range of possibilities. This is a realm full of shades of gray. It's a space of nonduality where the binary of *either-or*—"I am either intrigued by death or fearful of it"—gives way to *both-and*: "I am both curious to explore death and feel some anxiety about it."

The term "nondual" is a translation of the Sanskrit term "advaita," which means "not two" or non-separateness. That is, concepts can remain distinct while not being separate. They can exist simultaneously. Another related idea that is helpful here is that of the *dialectic*—when two things seem in conflict with one another, yet are revealed to both be true, for example, "I can prepare myself well for the end of life and prioritize living fully in the present." Anticipate an array of reactions to the exercises as your mood and mindset vary. By turning toward complexity, you can find harmony within it.

Value yourself. You are inherently worthy. You are deserving of respect and compassionate care. You have a lifetime of remarkable stories to share. If you were not raised to believe these things about yourself, allow this to be an opportunity to further develop your self-esteem. You are a work in progress with limitless potential, even in the moments you might doubt yourself or be most overwhelmed.

Being Enough

Doubts of *enoughness* regularly hinder people. *Am I prepared enough? Strong enough? Knowledgeable enough?* Partly, this stems from imposter syndrome, when people feel they don't measure up to others due to perceptions of inadequacy. I encourage those who grapple with these fears to be humble, ask questions, and stay open to learning, as those are the components of real wisdom. Try to lessen any pressure you might impose on yourself about how you "should" be, act, or feel due to external influences—the culture you were raised within, systemic oppression, and so forth—to reveal underlying truths. Strive to cultivate feelings of worthiness and courage.

Transform any rushes of insecurity into reverence for the work ahead. Tell yourself: *I worry because I care. I am concerned because this really matters to me.* That kind of messaging is self-compassion in action. It will help connect you, again and again, to yourself and your mortality.

CHAPTER 2

Connection

Compassion and connection go hand in hand. As part of our death wellness work, you are creating a compassionate space around and within you that feels personally affirming. This effort will reinforce the established, lasting connections you have to (1) your sense of self; (2) your reserves of strength; (3) your *source*, or what nourishes you internally; (4) your story, the narrative of your life; and (5) your supports, the resources you can draw upon—all supremely valuable attachments to forge.

Here are five opening questions to examine. You might sit with each for a minute or two. You might spend a brief amount of time writing down initial thoughts. Or you might simply skim them for now. We will be going into detail on each throughout the remainder of the book.

1. **Sense of self:** What relationship do you have with yourself?

2. **Strength:** What do you turn to when stressed?

3. **Source:** What sustains your inner well-being—your spirit or soul?

4. **Story:** What are your life chronicles?

5. **Support:** What resources—friends, family, care providers, and others—can you turn to for aid?

_____

_____

_____

_____

The Importance of External Connections

Humans are hardwired for connection. By nature, we are social creatures. Our brains are set up with mirror neurons that trigger facial expressions, reflecting what a listener is seeing and sensing from a speaker. This helps us read and respond to others, creating an "automatic, moment-to-moment resonance that connects us," as neurobiologist Amy Banks asserts. "People in our culture need to understand that healthy connection can reduce pain on all levels"—a powerful endorsement (Wellesley Centers for Women 2010).

Research by Richard Ryan and Edward Deci (2017) suggests that connection is one of three core needs that facilitate growth, enabling people to really thrive in life. The other two are autonomy (feeling in control of your own actions and decisions) and competence (feeling capable of achieving your goals). When robust in availability, these three components lead to optimal development and function. Each plays its own important role.

We can develop a sense of autonomy through meaningful activities that promote self-determination. Successful attainment leads to a sense of initiative as well as harmony between our inner self and life purpose. Conversely, when we feel controlled by external forces (rewards or punishments), it quells autonomy. Ultimately, both in good health and in sickness, many of us yearn to make significant choices for ourselves and to direct our care (self-determination). And by documenting care preferences, as you are within this workbook, you can add your voice to decision-making conversations—even for times when verbal communication might not be possible.

Competence is related to autonomy, yet distinct, as it describes our ability to cope with problems effectively and adjust ourselves and specific factors of a situation. When we attain feelings of competence, it encourages a sense of mastery. Ryan and Deci (2020) explain the need for competence is best satisfied within "well-structured environments that afford optimal challenges, positive feedback, and opportunities for growth." We can flourish, even during our final stage, when we feel we have a sense of agency over our remaining life and eventual death.

Finally, connection to others, or relatedness, rounds out the three needs. Here, what matters are interpersonal attachments and a sense of belonging within units (family, friend groups, and community). Forging close, caring relationships boosts psychological well-being, while deficient support can both hinder inner experiences and worsen harmful self-impressions.

When we cultivate them, connection, competence, and autonomy promote a substantive sense of purpose. They ignite our passion and satisfaction—our zest for life. People with high levels of drive and self-efficacy are better able to recognize meaningful reasons to live, and they continuously evolve in their thinking and behaviors.

Lack of Connection

What happens when these core needs aren't adequately met? In reality, the quantity and quality of our experiences and perceptions will fluctuate. Sometimes, we will feel empowered and validated. Other times, we will feel misunderstood or forgotten. You can probably think of areas of your life, whether in the present or in the past, in which you've been able to experience autonomy, competence, and connection. And you can probably also identify areas in your life where they have been lacking.

Perhaps by exploring lack of connection—or loneliness—in more detail, we can strengthen our resolve to better manage times of depletion while working toward replenishing our reserves. As discussed, death journaling is largely introspective work. And introspection is deeply personal. Even when working alongside others, our inner journey is solitary, which might feel lonely at times.

Loneliness

The antithesis of connection is loneliness—a rampant epidemic throughout the world. Even before the COVID-19 pandemic, social scientists named loneliness a major health concern. Geriatrician Carla Perissinotto defines social isolation as "an objective indicator of how much contact somebody has with other people," whereas loneliness is the subjective feeling of isolation (Ducharme 2020).

Being alone doesn't necessarily mean you're lonely, nor does being around people mean you're not. Loneliness is a particular sensation only the person experiencing it can really identify. The key difference between being lonely and being alone is emotional attachment, or connection. More definitively, being alone is a state of solitude, while loneliness is a perception. Loneliness can occur when we feel our true self is not being seen or understood by others or from within.

Loneliness can be fleeting or chronic. It is always personal though, meaning we experience it as a result of our interpretation of a situation. Social isolation clearly exacerbates it. Physical closeness does not always alleviate it. Some of us relish time alone, while others fear it deeply.

Loneliness Measures

If you feel inclined, take some time to assess your own level of loneliness as a way to gauge your capacity for mortality awareness practices. Answer the following questions, inspired by the University of California, Los Angeles (UCLA) three-item loneliness scale as well as the United Kingdom's Community Life Survey. You can choose to evaluate how you feel at present or how you have felt during the past week, month, year, or decade.

Ponder the following questions:

How often do you feel you lack companionship?

_____

_____

_____

How often do you feel left out?

_____

_____

_____

How often do you feel isolated from others?

_____

_____

_____

How often do you feel lonely?

_____

_____

_____

Contemplate and reflect on this sentiment widely attributed to Eda J. LeShan: "When we cannot bear to be alone, it means we do not properly value the only companion we will have from birth to death–ourselves."

_____

_____

_____

_____

_____

Reflections

How was that to assess loneliness? It may have felt disheartening or relieving or anything in between. Allow it to be whatever it was as you try to suspend any judgment. Your emotional state does not define who you are, nor will it necessarily last forever. As mentioned, loneliness is a common condition that many people experience. For most, it is transient and specific to circumstances. For others, it can become a spiraling cycle of thoughts and behaviors that magnify its intensity.

On the topic of loneliness, palliative care physician Robert Gramling writes, "I find that loneliness might be the single greatest source of suffering that seriously ill people encounter in our modern world. However, I am reminded daily that our most effective clinical tool for alleviating suffering is our interest in being fully present, of fearlessly bearing witness, of curiously wanting to know the person and, sometimes, merely offering space to laugh about...it all" (Arnoldy 2018, x).

While compassionate practitioners, like doulas and palliative care providers, utilize presence and attentiveness regularly, as individuals living our day-to-day lives, we do not always have immediate access to external support throughout challenging times. My questions, then, to you are: _Can you offer this type of thoughtful care to yourself? Can you extend and receive boundless self-compassion? Can you nurture connection?_

Cultivating Connection

How does it feel to be connected—to yourself, to others, and to the world at large? When we are lonely, we often feel adrift and sometimes lost entirely. We may also notice a physical sensation of heaviness or pain in our chest or gut. On the other hand, connection leads to contentment. It feels like returning home to a safe haven. This *home* is a warm, familiar place of refuge that provides security. It might not be one we have actually resided in or even visited, yet we can forge it within ourselves, the groundwork being self-compassion.

Through contemplation and practice, you can reinforce a sense of connection (internally and to your experiences) and carry it with you throughout upcoming explorations of who you are, what you fear, and any expectations you hold. First, take some time to consider what *connection* means to you as you complete the following exercise. Write freely as you consider the prompts.

Remember a time you felt truly connected. This could be the experience of a strong link to a supportive person or beloved companion animal, the natural world, your own sense of self, or a larger source. Describe the process of connecting and any associated feelings in detail.

_____

_____

_____

_____

_____

_____

_____

_____

Reflections

How was it to remember an experience of pure connection? How did it feel in your body? Did you notice any new or heightened sensations? What might this exercise illuminate in terms of your inner workings?

_____

_____

_____

_____

_____

Knowing what fostered this sense of connection you recalled, what might you seek out moving forward?

_____

_____

_____

_____

From the moment we are born until our last breath, connection enhances our health and happiness. During times of illness—and also when a person is dying—soothing, attentive treatment can bring needed comfort. Feeling the presence of those who care surrounding us can help relieve discomfort and unease whenever they might occur.

Later in the book, especially when you focus on drafting your end-of-life care wishes, you'll revisit the concept of interconnectedness in terms of identifying your circle of support and what layers you might need to add to it to complement what is available. But we mustn't lose sight of the one steady presence we can always count on—our own.

Innerconnectedness

Innerconnectedness is the unparalleled relationship you have to your wise self and inherent strength. Throughout this journey, you will continue to befriend yourself to experience innerconnectedness. Mortality awareness—the practice of acknowledging life's temporariness—will ask much of you, mentally and emotionally. Before reaching outward during intense moments, pause to reach in and see what's readily available. Consequently, you might find yourself opening more to the richness of solitude—aloneness free from loneliness—as you settle into a stance of anchored composure.

May this be a reclamation of your mortal being.

Part II

Preparedness: Opening to Death Wellness

When we retreat inward, we can begin to distinguish the enduring aspects of ourselves versus those that are more transient. What remains once we sort through passing moods or phases? Our fundamental essence or "core self" persists, as does the steadfast reality of our mortality. Our finiteness is a constant, try as we may to persuade ourselves otherwise.

As we wade through this complex topic, try to hold a few overarching questions in your mind: *Can death be an ally? Can I welcome mortality reminders, gently and regularly, into my awareness? What comes if I do? What comes if I do not?*

Mortality Salience

People who consider their own mortality and understand they will eventually die are said to have a mortality salience. Acknowledging the ultimate end of our physical self can produce anxiety. This is normal and expected. We are, like all animal beings, a species driven by survival. Even those among us who we feel have reconciled the inevitable can experience moments of angst when processing the reality of life's end. Throughout this part of the workbook, you will review strategies for interpreting and managing this most primal fear. As you begin, remember to choose the pacing and depth of your contemplation that feels best.

Mitigating Anxiety

To start, reflect on any healthy strategies you already utilize when dealing with stress or fear. Recall and describe reliable coping techniques you have used for soothing anxiety. List methods that have a proven record of improving your sense of wellness and creating calm.

_____

_____

_____

_____

_____

Reflections

How was that to think of your dependable tools? Did they come to mind swiftly, or was it challenging to name any?

_____

_____

Perhaps your collection is bountiful, or it might benefit you to spend more time brainstorming or practicing ways to nourish yourself. Focus on your physical, mental, and psychological needs. You might find solace in nature, movement, art, journaling, counseling, ritual, breath work, laughter, hobbies, friendships, or snuggling with a companion animal among other, countless ideas.

As an additional step, you might also think back on what hasn't worked well, including "quick fixes" (like numbing out with substances or devices) so you can attempt to avoid that pattern. Instead, have your trusty go-to approaches at the ready for any intense moments ahead.

Without courage we cannot practice any other virtue with consistency. We can't be kind, true, merciful, generous, or honest. —Maya Angelou

Nonexistence

Undeniably, it takes great courage to reclaim our mortality. When faced with the prospect of our ephemerality, or fleetingness, people commonly wonder: *How could it be that (someday) I will not be?*

Nonexistence is an unbelievable notion. In fact, our brains actively attempt to avoid internalizing this realization. Research shows the human mind goes to great lengths to shield itself from existential threat (Dor-Ziderman et al. 2019). Clearly, this is another tactic rooted in survivalism. In our logical minds, we know we will eventually die, yet our brains rework this as a phenomenon that happens either not at all, not for a very long time, or only to others.

How will you navigate this dissonance—this inner battle of contradictory thinking? This subjective disharmony? It's not always easy to sit squarely in mystery as we do when contemplating mortality. It is a space swirling with seemingly absurd certainties and unsolvable questions, and your space will be uniquely yours.

So, we need to have plenty of effective, accessible coping techniques. Highlight one or two examples that will be most apt for death journaling, either from your previous list of dependable approaches or you can brainstorm some new ideas.

_____

_____

_____

_____

CHAPTER 3

Mortality Awareness

When you think of life's end, what comes to mind? Much of the time, we don't evaluate our notions—the ones we hold as individuals or those we share within larger groups. By pausing to contemplate our perceptions of mortality—why we have them and where they came from—we can begin to decipher and question the validity of them.

Living and dying are concepts that defy any one explanation, making it challenging to answer the big question: *What is the purpose of existence?* "We're here to love," assert some people, while on the other end of the spectrum, others argue that humans are merely vessels for viruses and bacteria. Many religions and spiritual groups make claims regarding the "why" and "how" questions. And some people who narrowly escaped their demise (such as via near-death experiences) or who have returned from mystical experiences (for example, a psychedelic trip) have interpretations. Yet, they vary.

What's your current understanding, belief, or sense of what "life" is all about? And "death"?

_____

_____

_____

_____

_____

_____

Death as a Source of Anxiety

The adage "We fear what we don't understand" tends to pervade the weighty sphere of dying. The truth is, we cannot fully understand death, or even life, while we are alive—and that's our underlying human conundrum. As existential psychiatrist, Irv Yalom (2008, 1) suggests, human beings are "forever shadowed by the knowledge that we will grow, blossom, and inevitably, diminish and die." Yalom goes on to warn that death has the power to evoke feelings of powerlessness, separation, loss of control, and meaninglessness. For some individuals, the fear of death can go as far as to actually negate fulfillment and happiness.

In his book *The Denial of Death*, Ernest Becker theorizes that a biological need to control our fundamental death anxiety is in fact the basic motivation for all human behavior. He writes, "This is the terror: to have emerged from nothing, to have a name, consciousness of self, deep inner feelings, and excruciating inner yearning for life and self-expression—and with all this yet to die. It seems like a hoax… What kind of deity would create such complex and fancy worm food?" (Becker 1973, 87) Becker's stark messaging has numerous psychological and philosophical implications. These words could become fodder for fatalism, or they might lead us to speculate it's all random. They certainly beg the question, Why?

Why are we here? What is the point of it all?

Inspired by Becker's work, social psychologists Jeff Greenberg, Tom Pyszczynski, and Sheldon Solomon (1986) present the concept of "terror management theory" (TMT). TMT suggests people cope with existential terror by immersing themselves in cultural conceptions of reality—that is, certain worldviews—which offer meaning, purpose, and the hope of transcending death through literal or symbolic immortality. In short, people attempt to deal with death by trying to dodge it.

Many major religions, for example, afford "literal immortality" to followers with promises of an everlasting soul, heaven(s), afterlives, a "second coming," or reincarnation. Many societies offer ways to achieve "symbolic immortality" through being part of a "great nation," amassing wealth and possessions, noteworthy accomplishments, and having children (Ernest Becker Foundation n.d.). By relying upon literal immortality, we soothe our earthly concerns by believing there is *something more* after our physical body ceases to function. When striving for symbolic immortality, we try to project ourselves into the future by *making our mark* (creating art, writing books, procreating, and so forth) so our name might outlast our lifetime. These actions seem to lessen distress while keeping death at a distance.

How do these theories on death anxiety and terror management theory land with you? What are your impressions of literal and symbolic immortality? Give yourself a chance to assess and express any immediate reactions.

_____

_____

_____

_____

_____

A Balanced View of Mortality

In the face of mortal fear, are our efforts toward achieving literal or symbolic immortality negative, positive, or neutral? Perhaps "healthy" versus "unhealthy" might be better terms to ponder. Or maybe we can put aside the need to label or judge, and merely accept these tendencies as "expected" and "natural." Hundreds of studies have supported the theory that the awareness of life's end has the potential to create nervousness and compromise psychological well-being (Juhl and Routledge 2015). So, it seems important to explore our own response to the reality of mortality as we work through the pages of this workbook.

How have you reacted in the past to reminders of death—news of a loss, for example? TMT research finds one reaction to existential threat is to *other*, or to create distance from, those who threaten our illusion of invincibility. At the extreme, this can mean shutting out any mention of mortality and might even lead people to behave aggressively toward those outside of their belief system.

It can also take form in subtler ways. More commonly, we fish for details about a person's illness or cause of death to ease our own worries. I see this regularly in my deathcare work. For example, a person learns someone was diagnosed with lung cancer. A common follow-up question is, "Did they smoke?" If so, this provides relief if the person asking doesn't smoke because they feel less at risk for developing the disease. Or, if someone died of COVID-19, a person might want to know if the deceased had underlying medical conditions (namely, ones not shared). The closer an illness feels to us personally, the more it can threaten our perception of immunity.

If you weren't conscious of this tendency before now, you will likely notice it much more often. Sometimes, you'll witness others asking for specifics about an illness or death, and sometimes you'll find yourself digging for details. This is common. It doesn't need to be judged harshly—or necessarily avoided if the intent is to become a source of support as a listening ear. With increased awareness, you might find yourself needing less information than before, simply because you recognize the reason behind the probing questions.

As author and teacher, Pema Chödrön (2000, 40) explains, "The more we witness our emotional chain reactions and understand how they work, the easier it is to refrain. It becomes a way of life to stay awake, slow down, and notice."

Will you have moments of wanting to keep death at a distance? Yes, likely you will. We all do. As I pored over death terror research, I found myself feeling increasingly unsettled. Past losses reappeared as did current worries. I was flooded, and floored. As a deathcare worker and educator, life's end is never far from my thoughts. How could I have been caught off-guard? Well, because I am human. No matter how strong my practices are, I will feel unbalanced at times. Thankfully, I know these phases are temporary, and I can steady myself with mindful effort.

Keep in mind that you, dear reader, have chosen to explore your existence within the supported realm of this workbook. You are directing this journey—its depth and end goals. You will encounter challenges along the way, yet you are receiving numerous tools within these pages to maneuver through them. You are empowered to engage in death journaling in the ways you deem best.

Legacy Projects

As TMT research suggests, one way people can deal with mortal dread is to transcend it through immortality efforts. We can choose to interpret this as an invitation to immerse ourselves in meaningful work, thus transmuting any fear we may feel into thoughtful projects.

Legacy ("immortality") projects, when done with intention, can bring incredible beauty into the world. Some people start charities or annual fundraising events, while others create community gardens, knowing these efforts will outlast them. Some people fight for change in the form of revised legislation or rules. Others pass down priceless treasures, such as a secret family recipe, an artisan craft, or ancestral stories. Even simple acts of kindness or modeling embodied values can land you a prominent place in someone else's memory. Remembrance gifts, small and large, provide innocuous ways of projecting ourselves into the future while calming our nerves in the present moment.

For the sake of uncovering our greatest dreams, take some time now to think up your ideal legacy project and write about it in the following space. If money, time, and energy posed no constraints, what would you leave to your loved ones, community, or the greater world? What do you think would be most meaningful to you and others? Your idea can be outlandish, extravagant, or simple.

My dream legacy project:

_____

_____

_____

_____

_____

_____

_____

_____

_____

_____

_____

_____

Reflections

How was it to design your ultimate legacy offering? What would your hopes be for those who could enjoy what you imagined creating or gifting?

_____

_____

How does your creation reflect who you are and how you want to be known or remembered?

_____

_____

Even if your project seems entirely unfeasible, the details of the plan might speak to your virtues and values in ways that inform your mortality awareness practices.

Your entries throughout this workbook can become remembrance gifts you leave for those left behind. This is a healthy way to cope with the inevitability of the end of life. In the sections still to come, you'll find many more activities that will provide inspiration for expression. From quick messages to lengthy lists, your death journal will be replete with meaningful offerings.

If the reality of mortality ever feels overpowering, remember you can transmute that energy into goodness. Consider what you can generate and share with others—either loved ones or those (known or unknown to you) in the broader community.

Learning from Death Directly

As you ponder your place along the spectrum of death anxiety while keeping in mind that it's rarely fixed, you can begin to acknowledge how individual attitudes evolve partly from societal philosophies and practices. Many Western societies, in particular, perpetuate mortality aversion—people don't think about death except to consider how to avoid it. How did that happen?

How have so many of us living at this time separated ourselves so drastically from the natural order—the life cycle that encircles us all?

This widespread resistance to end-of-life matters stems partially from our neglected familiarity. As long as we have lived, we have died, although we used to accompany each other through the journey more often as kin. Even as recently as a few hundred years ago, people were raised seeing loved ones care for terminally ill relatives in the home. Family members washed and prepared their dead. Communities gathered for wakes and helped bury the deceased in simple plots. Due to forces like modernization and colonization, "caring for our own" has largely become a lost tradition.

In Europe, from the 1500s to the 1800s, life expectancy hovered between thirty and forty years. People died swiftly, and there were few interventions that might fend off an untimely demise, especially for those with infections or infants facing complications. During the 1800s, many Western cultures experienced significant changes influenced by societal shifts and advances in medicine. More people began receiving care in offices and hospitals, hygiene practices improved, and modern embalming practices began. Also, vaccines, medicines, and medical interventions became more available (in countries with wealth), staving off deaths caused by numerous communicable diseases.

All of this led to an outsourcing and medicalization of the end of life. Dying largely left our homes and hands, and fewer people regularly witnessed it as an expected part of our human existence.

Life and Death Perspectives

Think about your own childhood. Was the process of dying a regular part of life or kept at a distance? How was death explained to you? Without a doubt, your initial introduction to mortality left an indelible imprint.

_____

_____

_____

_____

_____

_____

How did loss itself first visit you? What theories, messaging, or beliefs do you carry as a result? Are they unshakable "truths" or malleable ideas? Take some time to reflect and write what comes to mind in the following space, including any lasting impressions.

_____

_____

_____

_____

Have you been able to share your personal experiences or perceptions with others? To reinstate and reinforce death literacy—knowledge of the dying process and deathcare system—we need to tell our stories and develop our understanding from hearing other people's accounts. In service of this, allow me to share my first experiences with the end of life.

The first time I sat close to the dying process was at age twenty-four when my aunt was terminally ill. Before getting sick, she had been so full of life with a true skip in her step. It was unfathomable to believe anything could slow her down, let alone rob us of her final decades, given she was only forty-nine. Pancreatic cancer, especially at that time, was a force well beyond the reach of medicine.

When my cousin called to let me know her mom had been admitted to the hospital and that I had better come quickly, I wasted no time. My coworkers sent me off with hugs. Before leaving home, I paused to write a quick note to my aunt—a farewell of sorts. I rolled it up and tucked it into the arms of a sweet stuffed bear she had given me months prior. I didn't have a clear plan for its use, but I thought it might act as a comforting and protective object—a talisman of sorts.

Soon, I was at the hospital in a room teeming with loved ones flanking my dear aunt, who undulated between groggy consciousness and sound sleep. Those of us in attendance did not know what to do with ourselves or this time. It felt strange as well as devastating. Later in the evening, fewer than a dozen of us remained. At this point, I followed my heart and asked for a few minutes alone with my aunt—a gift my cousins and uncle gave me without pause.

I carefully climbed onto my aunt's hospital bed, cuddled up against her weakened body, and unfurled the note I had brought. I read it aloud, voicing my gratitude for her loving, uplifting presence throughout my whole life. Though she could no longer open her eyes, she mustered the energy to whisper, "I love you." Mere hours after I left, a tear fell from her eye as she released into the mystery of death with her adult children and husband holding her hands.

I didn't have any frame of reference entering that experience or any formal guidance. I let things happen spontaneously—and I am forever thankful for those last moments of connection.

The first time I witnessed the moment of death was at age thirty-two when my grandfather was on hospice at home. Again, I entered with a mindset of openness along with some muffled worries, not knowing what to expect. My grandmother was exhausted from 24/7 caregiving, so she went to try to sleep knowing I would accompany my grandfather in her absence. I gathered my courage and sat close to my "Lelo" (for "abuelo," which means "grandfather" in Spanish).

He was already in his final sleep phase and did not appear to be in pain—no grimacing, moaning, or physical tension. The sight of him was quite shocking to me though. He had always been tall and thin, but he had lost substantial weight. His cheeks were hollowed, and his partially opened eyes looked glassy. He was lying on his side, and his body had drawn itself into the fetal position. His breathing was irregular, and his extremities were cooling as his system prioritized core functioning. I noticed each small detail as I received this last lesson from him.

I have heard people philosophize about dying. *What exactly is it? When does it start? When is someone living, and when are they dying?* I've heard some people equate the process with a type of labor, similar to the birthing process, because it seems to be work, requiring time and physical effort to complete. Many describe it as a transition, and that was certainly what I was observing.

My grandfather was technically alive, yet his body was clearly undergoing steady, incremental changes. He was there, yet he was unreachable. I wondered about his consciousness—if he had awareness and if he was maneuvering through this transition on a spiritual or emotional level. There was much to wonder about, but more importantly, to behold.

Those two losses greatly influenced my personal outlook on the end of life. Thankfully, they were well-supported passings. There wasn't significant suffering or agitation in either case. There are aspects of these deaths I hope to experience myself when it's my turn. I hope my pain will be managed well and any unease addressed. I hope to be surrounded by beloveds and soothed through this final endeavor. Not all deaths unfold in this same way though. Some are more complex than others. And it is probable death has visited you in various ways.

Have you had direct experience with the process of dying? If yes, what was that like? If no, how do you think that affects your outlook?

_____

_____

_____

_____

If your formative experiences of death were in any way sudden, that can be weighty to process. Unanticipated losses—those caused by violence, accidents, unforeseen conditions, or suicide—frequently involve compounding factors. There is no time to say goodbye. There is no chance to care for someone through their final moments. Shock combines with potential regret. Mourning is interrupted by unyielding questions: *Should I have known? Did I miss something? Could I have done something to prevent it?* Commonly, this type of grief is both acutely severe and long-lasting. Patience, along with holistic support—plus plentiful time for healing—is generally necessary.

It's also difficult to shift our focus back to ourselves and realize we cannot control everything about our own departure. Will it be unexpected? Anticipated? Quick or drawn out? Personally, I do find comfort, based on what I have seen and learned, in knowing death can be peaceful. Often, there are moments of beauty, grace, joy, and love—especially when people have had honest conversations with others ahead of time. Not always in every case—as there are no guarantees—but often enough for many of us who work in deathcare to build a solid measure of trust in the process. Hopefully, the work you do within and outside of this book helps bolster your sense of trust as well.

In the meantime, what goes unresolved can fester. And revealing your inner thoughts can be freeing. What questions about dying do you continue to hold? Concerns? Worries? Theories? Write to death directly and ask about all that occupies your mind at this moment.

Dear Death,

_____

_____

_____

_____

_____

_____

_____

_____

Reflections

How was that to pen a letter to death? Did it draw the notion of your eventual exit closer? Ultimately, when we invite death to join us as a quiet companion throughout our days, its presence might not feel quite so startling. As we bravely engage in death wellness practices—by considering our own perspectives on death or the legacies we might wish to leave behind—we might find ourselves prioritizing the time and energy we do have in ways that align with our values. Maybe then, the choices we make—from the mundane to the major—will be fueled by purpose more than fear.

CHAPTER 4

Memento Mori

Memento mori (Latin): remember death.

Death, our perennial certainty, has always been a part of life, and humans have always struggled to reconcile its inescapability. The practice of "memento mori" is thought to have started in early Roman times during ceremonial processions following victorious battles. A celebrated military leader would parade through packed streets on a chariot. Behind the leader would be an enslaved person whose sole responsibility was to whisper continuously, "Respice post te. Hominem te esse memento. Memento mori!" Translated, this means, "Look behind. Remember thou art mortal. Remember you must die!" The aim of the tradition was to keep the worshiped leader humble and aware of the transience of glory and existence at large.

Before then and since, other cultures, religions, and spiritualities have created similar visual and verbal nods to ephemerality. Ultimately, memento mori reminders can relieve some of our mortal fear by turning our attention to the time and opportunities we have in the present. What might contemplating memento mori make possible for you as you continue on your journey toward death wellness?

Remembering Death

Since entering the deathcare field, I haven't gone more than a few hours most days without thinking of my mortality. Sometimes, reminders—like a news story of a family saying goodbye to a beloved mother—strike me as heartbreaking. They hit close, and I think of the grief my loved ones would have experienced if the story had been ours. I imagine the world continuing to spin in my absence. I think of the projects I wouldn't have been able to complete.

Other times, paradoxically, I find myself feeling intrigued by life's end and yearn for the demystification that only death itself might provide. Mortal reminders also have the potential to energize and motivate me. My trusty mantra, "I'll never have more time than RIGHT NOW," urges me to embrace the current moment as it is the only one promised. Conversely, I sometimes feel bone tired and worn down by the suffering of the world, which prompts me to seek balance by pausing. You can't be passionately, robustly alive without also enjoying periods of deep rest.

I've come to practice a self-reminder of mortality at the end of each day, generally when saying good night to my kids or crawling into bed myself. I pause to acknowledge it is one less day in my grand total. I breathe that thought in and let it percolate as I ask myself: *Do I feel proud of today, or at least content with it? Did I leave anything unsaid or undone? Do I wish things had gone differently? What can I forgive within myself? What might I want to attempt or avoid tomorrow if I have the chance? What went well? What can I celebrate and appreciate?*

Symbolic Reminders

Beyond this nighttime ritual, I also scatter reminders throughout my home. In my office, I have a simple, handcrafted wooden casket that serves as a bookshelf until it's called to fulfill its ultimate purpose. As I write or teach, my eyes are regularly drawn to its contents. First, to a photo of my Aunt Nancy making one of her silly expressions I so dearly miss. It encourages me to not take myself too seriously. Next is a photo of my mom holding me as a baby. It reminds me how quickly time passes. Behind those frames, there is a painting of a tree in autumn that my daughter and I made together. It prompts me to acknowledge seasonality.

On the next shelf, I have two vision boards that nudge me to set and reach goals. The stuffed bear from my aunt with that rolled-up farewell message sits in front of a stack of poetry books I sometimes use for vigils. Scattered among the rest of the shelves, I have gifts made by my son, treasured childhood books, photo albums and scrapbooks, a talisman I crafted for my father-in-law when he was terminally ill, a painting of a sunset I worked on with a hospice client, and my death journal. Draped over it all is the dark blue "prayer shawl" a volunteer knit and gave to my Lelo for his time of dying.

Memento mori items evoke specific responses within us all. With the intention of incorporating death awareness practices to invigorate your energy for living well, what might you consider choosing as reminders? Will it be a token for your pocket, like the medallions of ancient Rome, some of which featured a skull for death, a tulip for life, and an hourglass for time? Or perhaps you'll wear a memento mori ring as people did during the Regency and Victorian eras. Will you display visuals inspired by *danse macabre* ("dance of death")—images depicting people, rich and poor, dancing with skeletons that emerged from the late Middle Ages? Or perhaps *Vanitas*, Dutch still-life paintings of the Baroque period that illustrated the fleetingness and vanity of life?

What calls to you?

Your mortality reminders can be obvious or understated so long as they signal you to awaken. For example, I have a necklace with my daughter's thumbprint from years ago that hangs close to my heart. What might you designate as your memento mori item(s)? What intentions will you set for their usage? Take some time to gather ideas, and then write about the process.

My memento mori symbols will be...

_____

_____

_____

_____

Their purpose is to...

_____

_____

_____

_____

_____

_____

_____

_____

Reflections

How do you envision utilizing memento mori symbols? How do you imagine their presence will affect your days? Is this a brand-new concept, or do you already have a practice established? If you regularly utilize memento mori symbols, can you find ways to strengthen your contemplation, perhaps in terms of frequency or intention?

_____

_____

_____

Here are some tips to consider as you either begin or deepen the practice of incorporating memento mori—reminders of death's inevitability and of life's beauty—into your daily life.

Incorporate reminders regularly, yet not obsessively. Behaviors can become routine with time and dedication, yet we must always seek to balance death reminders with living fully.

Set mental alerts. Make a plan to contemplate mortality regularly—when you awake, before sleep, or maybe during a midday break. Consistency fosters habituation.

Set calendar alerts. If mental alerts are not sufficient, consider scheduling in slots to pause and reflect. Make sure they are for times that are generally open or flexible.

Request additional signals from the universe or your divine source. Look beyond your concerted practice for examples and affirmation.

Now that I have been incorporating this type of mortality awareness for a while, I notice more everyday memento mori symbols all around. Contrast seems common. In my kitchen, I have a handful of thriving houseplants sitting on the ledge behind the sink. Above them resides a blackened petrified root my husband and I found while walking through the woods. I was immediately intrigued and enamored by its color and form. Outdoors, I'll often see a new sprout hiding behind a wilting blossom or the dried pods of last year's vegetation ensuring this year's crop.

They remind me: Life makes way for death makes way for life.

CHAPTER 5

Impermanence

Nothing stays the same, yet change can be virtually imperceptible when it's happening gradually. Children and baby animals, for instance, grow at unbelievable rates, yet the day-to-day shifts aren't terribly notice-able. And the lines on our faces and gray in our hair as we age sneak into our appearance slowly. Often, it's not until we see photos from different periods that we notice drastic transformations.

But again, from completely forgettable happenings to momentous events, nothing lasts forever. Moments are here, and then they're gone. Every sentient being will have its allotted lifespan. Even our sun is destined to eventually cease to exist, although perhaps not for billions of years. As humans, we have a cursory understanding of impermanence, yet we often base expectations on the notion that situations and relationships will continue on evermore. We might feel shocked and perhaps even wronged when things shift abruptly or come to an end.

Looking back on your days, how have you greeted change—as an uninvited visitor interrupting all you felt was predictable and constant? Or maybe as a guest offering some sort of gift or lesson? Likely, you've found yourself somewhere between those two extremes depending on the circumstances and your mindset at the time. Ultimately, when we're able to acknowledge the prospect of transitions and endings, we might find ourselves opening a bit more to the certainty of impermanence.

Recalling Our "Lasts"

When I feel particularly brave and nostalgic, I'll let myself think about "lasts." I'll recollect precious memories, such as the last time I visited my maternal grandparents' home before it sold—how it always smelled like my Lela's Chilean-Italian cooking and how the fabric wallpaper felt on my fingertips. Or I'll remember the last time I was on stage performing dance, hearing the roar of applause over the pounding of my heart. Or I'll reminisce about the last time I played "restaurant" or "trains" with my kids before they outgrew those imaginative games.

Do any "lasts" come to mind for you? If so, what do they make you think about? Do you feel fondness or a longing for times gone by? Or maybe a mixture of both?

_____

_____

_____

_____

_____

_____

For me, recalling "lasts" generates a self-imposed melancholy. Although some people might shy away from sentimentality, I have grown to appreciate the internal stirring that ensues. Sometimes I pine for the past. Other times, I soak in appreciation for having had an experience. Wherever my emotions land on the spectrum, I feel alive. "This is the *stuff*," I remind myself—not the things, but the stuff that really counts.

It's an aspirational goal I don't always successfully rise to meet, but instead of turning to synthetic thrills or numbing devices (such as driving too fast, mind-altering substances, or cell phones) to substitute or dampen natural emotions, I try to work with what life freely supplies—disappointments, delights, finales, and connections. I also invite those I support to reflect on these themes too.

Sometimes, this sort of reflection connects us back to moments and relationships that might otherwise go unexamined. Whether a person wishes to examine their past or not remains a personal choice though, of course. Once, when visiting a long-term hospice client, I asked about an old record player in the corner of the living room to entice him into conversation, knowing it might lead us down memory lane. He gave a brief response about converting the bottom to fit 78s before changing the topic. He wasn't interested in reminiscing.

However, the image of this piece of furniture remained in my mind long after I left. I wondered, *When was the last time it was played? Was it during an ordinary weekday dinner or maybe on a special occasion? Was it a sad or happy song? Classical music? A pop hit?* Most pressing on my mind: *Did anyone have any inkling it would be the very last time an album would be played on it, its swan song?*

Do you feel open to further exploring your "lasts"? If so, read the following poem and then reflect on the prompts to follow.

"On Joy and Sorrow," by Gibran Kahlil Gibran (1923)

Then a woman said, Speak to us of Joy and Sorrow.

And he answered:

Your joy is your sorrow unmasked.

And the selfsame well from which your laughter rises was oftentimes filled with your tears.

And how else can it be?

The deeper that sorrow carves into your being, the more joy you can contain.

Is not the cup that holds your wine the very cup that was burned in the potter's oven?

And is not the lute that soothes your spirit, the very wood that was hollowed with knives?

When you are joyous, look deep into your heart and you shall find it is only that which has given you sorrow that is giving you joy.

When you are sorrowful look again in your heart, and you shall see that in truth you are weeping for that which has been your delight.

Contemplate Gibran's words for a few moments before continuing.

Now, think back on any prominent "lasts" from your life. They might include actual goodbyes or the last time you saw someone. It might be the last time you did something special. It might be your final day at a job, school, or home you loved. Write about what is most memorable from those times.

_____

_____

_____

_____

_____

_____

Reflections

How was that to contemplate what has passed? Was it touching to reflect on these "lasts"? Did it open you up to feel the power of these experiences, or did it lead you to sadness and a need to turn away from the memories? Did it stimulate an array of emotion? What will you carry forward from this exercise? Will you notice *lasts* more often?

_____

_____

_____

_____

Marking the Moment

Sometimes, we're able to know it'll be the last of something, and we might be able to create a way of commemorating it. People with terminal conditions who have reached a place of acceptance with their prognosis might want to plan certain events as part of their final wishes. This might include one last trip to the seashore or one last gathering of all living relatives. It might mean returning to the market they worked at during younger years or traveling to a place they have always wanted to visit.

Before supporting people as a doula, I assumed I would react to receiving a terminal diagnosis by (1) immediately railing against it and then (2) drafting my "bucket list" (as in, what I hope to accomplish before "kicking the bucket"). Now, I'm not so sure. The end of life is a time rife with complexity. A person's energy steadily decreases as they near death, and there are sometimes uncomfortable side effects caused by treatments or the disease process itself. Moreover, there are endless medical appointments and equally endless decision-making points competing for a person's attention.

If you're facing an illness or a diagnosis, you might wonder about questions like:

- Do I get a second (or third) opinion?

- Do I continue with curative treatments?

- Should I consider clinical trials?

- Do I accept palliative care to address pain and suffering?

On more practical or metaphysical levels, you might ask:

- Do I remain living at home or move elsewhere?

- Are my affairs in order?

- Have I selected a proxy, surrogate, or agent who can advocate for my preferences if or when I no longer can?

- What will happen to my dear pet(s) and all my belongings?

- What preparations can I make now to ensure my loved ones aren't overly burdened later?

- What conversations do I need to have, and what work do I need to complete?

Given all these complicated lines of inquiry, my own perspective has evolved. The end of life is perhaps not the ideal time to launch an extensive bucket list tour! Instead, I now aim to regularly address and complete preparatory work instead of either (1) shielding myself from the inevitable or (2) stockpiling grandiose projects for that final period. I try to plan what I can in advance and have important conversations about what matters most with who matters most. And I strive to make my bucket list ambitions a reality while I have the time and energy while admitting that a lifetime might always feel too short no matter how long it is.

You are arriving to this workbook at your own current status. Perhaps you're thinking about these matters before facing a serious medical episode. Or perhaps death is a more immediate possibility. Either way, it's never too early or too late to either begin or revisit these topics. Take a few minutes to think about your own bucket list, whether you have one established already or not. Write what comes to mind.

My bucket list...

_____

_____

_____

_____

_____

_____

_____

Reflections

Can you carve out time and resources now to fulfill any of these goals? Are there some that seem lofty or unreachable? Are there others that are more attainable? Does it make sense to prioritize and rank them?

When it comes to the more practical questions mentioned previously—like getting your affairs in order and making necessary, pragmatic preparations for the end of life—see the resources within in the appendices for more information.

_____

_____

_____

The Art of Goodbye

In addition to reaching for goals and bucket list dreams, we can also prepare for our final phase of life, whenever it may come, by practicing the art of goodbye. Instead of allowing ourselves to rush through endings, we can try to commemorate times of transition.

Of course, this is not an easy prospect because new beginnings are alluring. They're packed with intrigue and promise. For most of us, it is much more appealing to focus on what's next in lieu of paying attention to what has passed. But this temptation keeps us from experiencing the full gamut of what life offers. When we protect and distract ourselves from sadness and complexity, it leaves us ill-prepared for major change. Perhaps, if we can begin acknowledging small-scale endings along the way, we will be better able to handle more profound ones in the future.

Years ago, my family started a tradition of marking significant endings and beginnings with "blessing stones." When our sweet dog Bella died, we all took part in her farewell. My kids were quite young, and I wanted to make sure they were involved in ways that felt okay. First, we each set off to find a special gift from nature—often a stone, but it could also be a pinecone, flower, leaf, or anything else—and then we gathered around the grave my husband had dug on the edge of our yard. We took turns holding out our simple gift in outstretched hands while filling it up with memories, words of thanks, and wishes for Bella. We dropped in our blessings along with some tears. It was a simply orchestrated way to process and heal.

There's no strict definition of what makes a transition "significant," but I've continued to incorporate blessing stones when a particularly special or notable time is coming to a close or when one is starting. During the initial summer of the COVID-19 pandemic, I escaped with my family to my grandparents' lake house for a week. We had been stuck at home so much during lockdowns that a change of scenery was amazing. Days stretched on with rounds of swimming, board games, books, and cooking over an open fire with the sunset glistening on the water. At the time, we were enjoying a temporary reprieve from high viral caseloads, so some relatives and a few friends came to visit. All-in-all, it was magic—low-stress and exactly what we needed to recharge.

As our last day approached, our hearts grew heavy. During our final morning, in the middle of packing and cleaning, sadness was giving way to crankiness. I hated the thought of leaving such a beautiful experience with such negative attitudes. I knew we needed to lean into the sadness. We had to give our feelings space to breathe. So, I pressed pause on the task list and asked the family to gather blessing stones and meet me on the dock.

Once gathered, I asked everyone to think of their favorite moments from the week we had together. We took turns filling up our blessing stones and sharing:

Drinking our morning coffee and tea on paddleboards while the sun came up. Jumping on the water trampoline with friends. Making fires. Having s'mores. Playing frisbee. Reading comics. Watching old cartoons. Eating smoked cheddar cheese and pepperoni. Seeing loved ones. Getting treats from the ice-cream boat.

Memories flowed, and then we dropped, threw, or skipped our stones into the lake. We found that by reviewing highlights and bringing gratitude into focus, we were able to carry forward some of that bliss we had enjoyed. Of course, our hearts still ached a little as we returned to normal life, but bittersweetness can be confirmation of a time relished. Joy and sorrow go hand in hand.

Have you had a similar experience? Are there rituals you and your family or friends have used to mark the end of something or the passing of time? Are there traditions you might want to establish now?

_____

_____

_____

_____

When, Not If: Accepting the Inescapable

When we're not accepting of changes or endings, we tend to engage in magical thinking. I have a relative who refuses to say, "When so-and-so dies," and instead says, "If." Logically, she knows this is wishful, yet the prospect of a devastating loss leads her to try to subdue reality.

Death can feel like the ultimate enemy. It's completely unacceptable even though it is inescapable. How can we cope?

One way might be to introduce mortality awareness through the language we use—into the conversations we have with others and the stories we share. Many of us, especially those of us who spend any time with youth, have opportunities to share what we know with those who are younger than us—maybe in response to questions they have or maybe to help prepare them for situations they might face. Death is, of course, one such situation.

When my paternal grandfather died, for instance, my children were in elementary school, and people expressed varying opinions about whether to include them in the process. With thoughtful planning, we decided to invite them to participate to the degree they preferred. They asked questions—some existential, others practical. Some I could answer, while in response to others, I could only join them in bewilderment. I chose not to pretend to know everything. Instead, we worked through unanswerable issues and big feelings together with open communication.

The afternoon of Gramp's wake, we talked about what to expect: an event at a place we had never been before that looked sort of like a house with a few living rooms inside; a large gathering of people; a mostly quiet time with some music playing in the background and a slideshow of photos on loop; some tears and hugs; and, most notably, Gramp's body laid to rest in the wooden casket they had seen their great uncles building. I explained he would look very peaceful, but that he wasn't asleep. His body had stopped working. His heart wasn't beating, and he was no longer breathing. Gramps had died. I let them know they could go up and say goodbye to him if they wanted, but they didn't need to decide in advance.

Fortunately, they were able to have a designated person (my mom, their "Nana") who offered to look after them and was willing to leave when they decided it was time. This way, I could also connect with family members I didn't see often, knowing the kids had steady support and an exit plan. In the end, they came and observed, visited, and developed a frame of reference for loss. They said farewell to Gramps and placed simple, love-filled gifts (blessing stones) by his clasped hands. And I had the opportunity to prepare them as best I could for what they'd encounter and to be there for them as they encountered it.

How about you? What sorts of conversations have you had with those you love about death—or times of great transition and change in general?

_____

_____

_____

If you haven't had many opportunities for this, which sorts of conversations about death or other times of great change might you like to have with those around you?

_____

_____

_____

Of course, there's no one right way to introduce children, or anyone, to this final part of life, yet I would argue we have a moral imperative to prepare and support one another earlier and with more intention. This way, for the generations to come, people will become more death literate.

Because of my doula work, my kids know birth and death, but what I've done with them isn't outside the range of what anyone can do with the children in their life or anyone else they care about. I try to broach complex topics in response to my kids' curiosity, to what life presents, and to what I know will occur eventually—hopefully without overwhelming them. As a result, we have experienced a range of emotions together, including anticipatory grief. This can be heavy, yet we are allowing strong feelings to surface within the warmest of embraces.

I also make sure to remind them: coming to terms with mortality does not mean we need to be happy about it.

Death Positivity

Popularized by mortician Caitlin Doughty, "death positivity" became a movement to normalize dying in the same way the "sex positivity" movement has encouraged healthy discourse about human sexuality. As explained on Doughty's site, The Order of the Good Death (n.d.), "People who are death positive believe that it is not morbid or taboo to speak openly about death. They see honest conversations about death and dying as the cornerstone of a healthy society."

Although the term "positive" is used, it does not mean people need to be pleased with the reality of life's end. We do not need to eagerly await death's arrival or welcome it with open arms in order to make space for its eventuality. We don't need to disregard feelings of despair or anger when we're reeling from loss.

Our relationship with mortality can fluctuate, just as with any enduring relationship. Depending on our emotional bandwidth, we might have time spans during which we try not to acknowledge death. There might be other phases when we step closer to the topic, inspired by intrigue or faith. Maintaining a long-lasting, yet flexible awareness of our mortality not only grounds us in the moment, but it also prepares us for times of liminality.

Liminal Space

Amid any transition, there's a starting place and an ending point. Liminal space is what connects the two. It's the space between. Many changes in life, both expected and unanticipated, feature this progression—birth and death most strikingly. Throughout my years of being a doula, I have noticed how uncomfortable people can be with liminality.

Life presents many of these drawn-out "in-between" times. The journey of pregnancy is a sort of liminal space. Simply put, there's a nonpregnant person who then becomes pregnant who then is no longer pregnant. Altogether, it's a colossal transition; broken down, it's a million miniscule changes. The liminality that first caught my attention, though, was during the throes of active labor.

The pushing phase is an extreme, condensed example of liminal space. The body goes through extraordinary upheaval with hormone surges and physiological urges. This is when I have observed remarkably varied reactions from those witnessing the process. Some people are able to stay calm, centered, and trusting. They can sit on their hands. They can "watch and wait." They can simply *be*. This can include support people as well as nurses, midwives, and obstetricians.

Others find this part of birthing absolutely unbearable. They have to *do something*—anything. They fill any quiet with noise. They direct and instruct instead of allowing the laboring person to listen to their body. Of course, intervention is sometimes necessary and lifesaving, yet even during straightforward cases, this need to act persists in some people.

After noticing these variations, I thought more about why this discomfort might arise. Although some nerves might be rooted in lack of comprehensive training or exposure to "normal" birthing or might be a result of imprints from prior difficult experiences, I theorize the main culprit is people's acute discomfort with suffering. We tend to shield ourselves from it. We generally turn away, not knowing how to respond or fearing we will make things worse. Or we try to hurry up and get past tough times.

I've seen this tendency at the end of life too. A prominent example of liminal space is when someone is anticipating the possible confirmation of a serious diagnosis or answers about treatment options. This waiting period can be brutal. Dealing with the unknown can be gut-wrenching. It's not uncommon for people to say that once they *knew* what they were dealing with, they felt relief, even when the news itself was devastating.

Another type of liminal space occurs during active dying. At this time, there is often less to do. People no longer need drinks or food, which is a particularly heart-rending shift because many people offer care through nourishment. During this phase, a person who is terminally ill is generally no longer as responsive or able to work on legacy gifts—like final letters—for loved ones. There will be sporadic personal care tasks or medication administration, yet it is quieter. Time slows. Caregivers and visitors begin to realize it is the final stage. Anticipation swells as the end nears, and the promise of finality materializes.

During these moments, I might gently encourage others to lean into what is happening, calmly noting changes in regard to the dying process and what they might mean, while recognizing people's differing levels of comfort. I might offer ideas for continued connection and invite people to speak directly to their person. I might invite them to share treasured memories or stories.

This is not a time that needs to be filled with trivial busyness or planning for "after." There will be long days to come with a void left by the loss. Right now, the moments can be devoted to presence—to really experiencing and understanding what's going on, as best we can.

Have you experienced this type of liminal space, laden with mystery?

_____

_____

_____

_____

Have you found yourself turning away from liminality to spare yourself discomfort? If so, please know it is a common reaction to hardship. As you continue to develop knowledge of the end-of-life domain, you might also cultivate courage to face what feels unbearable yet inevitable.

Navigating Liminal Space

Liminal space, or the "in-between phase" when time slows, is best understood within the broader framework of a rite of passage—a ritual, event, or experience that marks or constitutes a major milestone or change in a person's life (Merriam-Webster.com Dictionary, s.v. "rite of passage").

Anthropologists have identified various rites of passages, including birth and death, across history and cultures. They feature three common components:

1. Severance

2. Threshold

3. Incorporation

Severance is the tipping point. A person beginning a rite of passage must separate themselves from old ways and prepare to enter the unknown. The organization Rites of Passage (2015), which leads wilderness quests, describes it as "the phase of preparing to leave everything behind, gathering together in soul and body just what you will need for your journey." When a person who is terminally ill reaches this "tipping point," they sometimes feel an urgency to "nest," just as expectant parents sometimes do. This flurry of activity might include cleaning, organizing, and readying themselves, their home, and their beloveds for what is to come.

Threshold is the liminal space that follows severance and precedes whatever transformation is to come. It's the space *between worlds* where you let go of old ways yet haven't quite established new ones to rely upon. In childbirth, again, it includes pregnancy, labor, and delivery. As for death, the threshold is when the end draws near and people transition into active dying and retreat inward. They spend more time sleeping and, even when awake, seem distant almost as though they're in another realm. To caregivers, it sometimes feels like their person is pushing them away. Really, this is a natural part of the journey as the traveler progresses into depths unreachable by others.

Incorporation is a person's reemergence in a new state. It means integrating all the hard-won insights from the quest. In birth, this would happen after delivery when a person takes on the role of parent to the new baby. In death, people have a variety of hopes or beliefs about what, if anything, comes next. We can also understand this phase in terms of those left behind after somebody dies (the "survivors"). Their perspectives have undoubtedly changed, and they might feel utterly shattered. The process of piecing together their new identity and making sense of an altered world is a substantial part of incorporation and of healing while grieving.

Do you acknowledge or honor rites of passage in your life—events like new beginnings, endings, births, or deaths? If so, are these traditions rooted in your culture, religion, or spirituality? Or are they ones you have developed in other ways? And if you haven't done much to commemorate rites of passage, might you want to consider introducing these types of traditions more formally?

_____

_____

_____

Integrating Impermanence

As you deepen your death wellness practice by incorporating some of the concepts covered in this part of the workbook, such as memento mori and impermanence, here are some sentiments to keep in mind: Linger, don't cling. Savor delight and connection. Embrace what makes you smile.

Then, remember you can never repeat an experience in the exact same way. It's powerful to allow any poignant, sorrowful feelings to rise while reminiscing about times gone by. Memories can both create and soothe a sense of longing.

How might you add reminders of impermanence into your regular life?

You could work on a jigsaw puzzle. Put it together piece by piece (a meditative process itself). Once finished, pause to celebrate your accomplishment, and then take it all apart. Another idea, if it's possible, is to build a sandcastle at the ocean's edge during low tide. Stand back to enjoy your creation, and then watch the waves pull your artistic work back into the sea. Lastly, you could make a nature mandala with any supplies you can find around your home or in a nearby park. Use fallen sticks, pieces of bark, pinecones, and flowers to build an outer frame and inner design. Bask in your creativity, and then walk away knowing nature will make use of what you made.

Remind yourself: Fleetingness does not diminish significance. Just because something cannot last does not mean it didn't matter.

What will you try over the next few weeks to give yourself a small, tangible experience of impermanence?

_____

_____

Once you've completed the practice you've chosen, come back to the book and jot down a few notes about the experience. What was it like? What did it teach you? How did it make you feel?

_____

_____

_____

Another quality you can strive to bring to your life is *equanimity*: mental or emotional stability or composure, especially under tension or strain; calmness; equilibrium (dictionary.com, s.v. "equanimity").

Just as a well-rooted tree can sway in strong wind and weather fierce storms, we too can ground ourselves firmly. This is not to say we should remain stiff and unyielding. Circumstances will cause us to flex and, at times, bend significantly. In such times, we strengthen our resolve to stay open to whatever may come by remembering the guarantees of liminality, impermanence, and our mortality. Healthy death awareness does not mean hyper-focusing or obsessing about endings. It means gradually coming to terms with reality while also concentrating on the potential of the present moment.

How will you try to bring equanimity into your day-to-day life? What imagery or reminders might reinforce your practice?

_____

_____

Your "Why"

Finally, we turn to the last concept we'll explore in this chapter, as your understanding of impermanence and death wellness continues to evolve: your purpose.

Ultimately, life is an endless series of mostly dull moments strung between sporadic, pivotal events. And most of us enjoy a humble existence. Your purpose for living doesn't need to be complex or elaborate. Fame and fortune do not equal meaning. Some of us *know* what we are meant to be or do during our tenure on Earth. Some marvel at possibilities without identifying any in particular. Others might not ever ask themselves such a philosophical question.

Your reasons for living might be obvious and unshakable, or they might seem more elusive. Wherever you are in the continuum of knowing your purpose, focus your attention on this inquiry: What is your *why*? Then, write about it in the following exercise.

My *why*

I am here to: _____

_____

_____

I aspire to: _____

_____

_____

I dedicate myself to: _____

_____

_____

Reflections

How was it to consider your purpose in life? Weighty? Illuminating? Have you been living in alignment with your *why*, or might you make changes to do so?

_____

_____

_____

Hopefully identifying goals fosters more inspiration than frustration.

It's kind to offer ourselves healthy margins. Just as we wouldn't expect a beloved to be perfect, we won't always act as our most authentic selves. Also, we don't need to always be serious. Living well means opening to it all, which includes fun! When you want to keep it light, give yourself permission to do so. When you are depleted, nurture yourself. Guilt isn't a great motivator—mortality awareness can be, though.

In the end, a healthy regard for impermanence, liminality, equanimity, and purpose leaves us with the following knowledge—a dialectical sort of truth: time passes, yet this moment is mine.

Part III

Pause and Practice: Strengthening Your Coping Techniques

Generally—but especially during times of stress, including serious illness and anticipatory grief before a major loss—anxiety can lead to problematic physical and emotional manifestations. These can include elevated blood pressure and heart rates, and even mental health conditions. Dame Cicely Saunders, a founder of formal hospice services, understood the connection between the mind and body. She coined the term "total pain" to describe the physical, psychological, social, emotional, and spiritual elements of suffering in seriously or terminally ill patients. The potential occurrence of pain and suffering makes it imperative for care providers—and anyone, really—to prepare themselves well with specialized tools.

In this section, we'll explore some coping techniques you can use in difficult moments—while working through end-of-life planning here or during future moments of struggle. Practicing these techniques will help you meld together many of the ideas you've read about so far: innerconnectedness as well as compassion—for yourself and others alike. It'll also be a meaningful addition to your death journal, and it may become a vital component of your *deathcare plan*.

Meeting Pain with Presence

During one shift as a hospice volunteer, a nurse asked if I could sit with a resident (whom we'll call Jonathan) while they adjusted his medication. The nurse explained Jonathan was struggling with breathlessness exacerbated by anxiety. Other than that, I knew nothing about this person I was about to meet, which is actually my preference because I would rather enter into the interaction as open as possible.

I paused at his doorway to take a few "threshold breaths," releasing what I was carrying and steadying myself for what was ahead. After Jonathan answered my knock with a quiet "Come in," I was immediately struck by how homey it felt inside. Artwork and memorabilia lined the walls and leaned against the coffee table. There were numerous musical instruments scattered about. This place had been personalized—an effort I always suggest clients consider, whether they are preparing for birth or death, so care providers will remember that an individual inhabits the space.

Jonathan was perched on a tripod stool, hands clutching his thighs, alternating between leaning forward and trying to stretch his torso upright. Clearly, he was uncomfortable. "Jackie"—his nurse—"is working on your meds," I conveyed, hoping the update might bring some relief. "Can I sit with you while you wait?" Jonathan nodded and gestured toward a nearby chair. I gingerly lowered myself down while slowing my breath.

What now?

I didn't know this person. We had no rapport built. I wondered if it would be awkward to hold absolute silence. I didn't want to make him use any extra breath on small talk though. I scanned the room in genuine amazement and decided to trust my instincts. "This artwork is incredible," I began, noting the colors and textures. "Please don't feel like you need to speak," I followed up. "Truly." Jonathan mustered a faint smile.

I asked a few yes-or-no questions so he could simply nod and continued to stay calm in my movements, expressions, and breathing pattern. A turkey outside the window caught my eye. It was a lone male bird, fairly large in size, rolling in the garden soil and shaking out its feathers. I provided commentary to Jonathan, who had begun responding in short sentences. "That was inspired by a trip out West," he then said, returning our attention to the first painting I had noticed.

By the time the nurse came into the room, probably about ten minutes had passed. Jonathan was now strumming his guitar, playing me an original song that he had composed. I was entranced. The sight surprised the nurse who had clearly been rushing to come to her patient's rescue. Jonathan's breathing had regulated, and he was no longer scared from air hunger. He chose to take the medicine anyway as a preventative measure. We were all relieved he was doing better.

Jonathan had been trapped in a brutal cycle of oxygen deprivation caused by the progression of his disease, which led to anxiety, which led to irregular breathing that worsened his distress and fear. By offering him distractions through presence and conversation, I invited Jonathan to turn his focus elsewhere, allowing for a slight reprieve. Even during tense moments such as these, we can often harness and direct the course of a distress cycle, either toward crisis or stability.

The relationship between thoughts and sensations is undeniable. Relaxing the mind can often help relax the body. This is especially crucial while navigating the end of life—whether you're supporting someone through it, preparing for it, or navigating through the actual experience of it yourself.

CHAPTER 6

Relaxation Exercises

In a study on relaxation exercises, researchers Samantha Norelli, Ashley Long, and Jeffery Krepps (2021) explain how feelings of stress can include physiological responses, such as increased heart rate, shortness of breath, and muscle tension, along with the subjective emotional experience. Relaxation techniques can aid in the reduction of these symptoms. Approaches such as breathing exercises, progressive muscular relaxation, guided imagery, and visualizations can be effective at decreasing distress and relieving unease.

Your breath-word visualization from the beginning of the book is a simple example of a relaxation exercise. You can also utilize a mantra or favorite line from a poem or prayer in place of your special word. You can breathe a sentence in and then mindfully release any tension with a whispered "haaa" as you exhale. The options for customization are endless.

As a doula, I'm fascinated by people's varying levels of openness to these techniques. Some love to set off in their imagination as I guide them on a mental excursion. Others are reluctant and get stuck in their logical minds, blocking their visions from taking over. It's always an enlightening process, however it unfolds, and can offer clues about unique preferences. Let's try two exercises together now.

Passive Muscle Relaxation: A Coping Technique for Stress, Suffering, or Sleeplessness

Passive muscle relaxation involves visualizing your body in detail and relaxing each part. This can be particularly helpful if you tend to have a lot of aches and pains, in addition to muscular tension. First, ask yourself how tense and stressed you feel. On the line below, mark your current stress level.

Maximum stress   **Medium stress**   **No stress**

Find a quiet, comfortable place to practice. For this exercise, it's best to lie down, with your hands at your sides if that's comfortable for you. Read over the entire technique a few times, so you don't have to refer to the book repeatedly as you practice. Or you can choose to record yourself reading the script aloud in advance of sessions.

To begin, focus your awareness on your breath. Feel the air enter your body, guided by the rising of your belly. Feel the air being eased out as your belly falls.

Do this three times, then close your eyes, if comfortable.

Bring to mind a soothing color. It can be white, yellow, blue, or any color that's soothing for you.

Imagine that this color is in a ball at the soles of your feet. Spend some time feeling the light from this ball shining in the room. Imagine that this light radiates relaxation and well-being.

Imagine this light entering your body through the tips of your toes, feeling your toes relaxing.

Imagine the light traveling up through your feet and radiating down into your heels, and then into your ankles. Imagine your feet being filled with relaxing light, perhaps feeling a bit heavier (more grounded).

Imagine the light traveling through your shins and calves, relaxing your muscles as it goes. Moving slowly upward, imagine the light relaxing your knees, your thighs, and into your torso, relaxing all the muscles along the way.

Imagine this relaxing light beginning to travel up your back, relaxing your spine. Feel the contact between your back and the surface beneath you.

Imagine the relaxing light bathing all the internal organs in your core, relaxing even deeper as you send light throughout your middle section.

Imagine this light infusing and relaxing your lungs and growing brighter as you belly breathe.

Imagine your heart pumping this relaxing light through every vessel in your body.

Imagine the light filling and relaxing your chest.

Now imagine that the relaxing light enters your body through the tips of your fingers on both hands. Imagine it slowly moving upward through your hands and wrists, relaxing the muscles as it moves. Feel it moving upward, relaxing your forearms and elbows. Imagine it continuing to move upward, relaxing the muscles all the way up to your shoulders.

Imagine that the light relaxes your neck and your throat, and then your chin and jaw. Imagine the light relaxing your cheeks, your tongue, and your nose. Feel it infusing and relaxing your eyes and eyelids, then your ears, then your forehead, and finally up through the top of your head.

Now imagine that the light has filled your entire body. Feel the light growing more relaxing with each breath. Sense it getting brighter with each breath—each time you inhale, each time you exhale.

Now imagine that the light begins to travel down through the top of your head, rejuvenating you, sweeping away all stress and tension, and wiping away any physical discomfort or pain. Imagine that all that is left in the place of any unpleasant physical sensation is relaxation and light.

Imagine your head and face being loosened, relaxed, and refreshed as the light moves down; then imagine your neck and shoulders being wiped clean of any tension or stress.

Imagine your chest, back, and all the bones and organs of your torso being relaxed, rejuvenated, and refreshed as the light moves down.

Feel it loosening and rejuvenating your shoulders, then your upper arms, and then your forearms. Imagine the light slowly moving down into your wrists and then your hands, loosening and rejuvenating them.

Moving slowly down through your legs, imagine your thighs, your knees, and then your lower legs being relaxed, rejuvenated, and refreshed as the light moves farther down.

Imagine your ankles, your heels, and your feet being loosened up, all the way down through your toes.

Now imagine that the light goes back into a ball underneath your feet. The light is as bright as the sun. Know that it is there any time you need it. All you need to do to access this wonderful, natural feeling of relaxation is to breathe through your belly, become aware of the light beneath your feet, and feel it infuse your body.

Be aware of how your body feels as you rest in this relaxed state.

If you feel that you haven't experienced enough of an effect, repeat the exercise. Pay close attention to each muscle group along the way on both sides of your body.

When you're ready, gently open your eyes. Wiggle your fingers and toes. Gently roll your body over to one side. Get up slowly.

After completing the passive body scan, mark your stress level on the line below.

Maximum stress   **Medium stress**   **No stress**

(This exercise was adapted from "Mindfulness for Prolonged Grief" by Kumar et al. 2013.)

Reflections

How do you feel after completing this relaxation exercise? How is your inner self (mind and spirit)? And your outer self (body)?

_____

_____

_____

Are you enjoying a greater sense of calm? Have you released tension?

_____

_____

_____

Are there any words or phrases that might work better for you? If so, cross out what doesn't resonate and make edits within your workbook for your next practice.

Next, we'll try a detailed visualization exercise.

Visualization Exercise: Your Special Place

You'll want to set aside about ten to fifteen minutes for this practice, including a reflection period at the end. First, find a quiet, restful place. Review the following script and tips a few times and then talk yourself through the process when you're ready, or you can record yourself reading the script and play it back.

Even if you have done similar visualizations in the past, activate your curiosity to see what might be new this round. If you're feeling skeptical—maybe you've tried this sort of exercise before and didn't enjoy it—give this activity a chance to either surprise you or confirm your opinion. Generally, people have positive experiences with these types of exercises. But if you become anxious or feel unsafe at any point, you can bring yourself back to the present moment and practice self-nurturance as needed.

Relax your breathing and settle into your body. Find as much comfort and ease as possible. Continue to slow your movements and soften any tension you're experiencing. Turn your attention inward as you breathe in relaxation.

In your mind, picture yourself curled up comfortably on a bed of fluffy cushions. Take a few more breaths and enjoy this peaceful tranquility. Now see yourself beginning to unfurl, feeling refreshed and ready to venture.

As you raise your head, you see a lush expanse of deep green grass in front of you. It's soft and warm under your feet, and you feel called to follow where it leads. Along the edge of the path, you see colorful blooms and butterflies. All is peaceful and quiet here. There's a gentle breeze that smells of your favorite flower. As you continue walking on the grass, feel the sunshine warming your skin.

You are nearing the end of the pathway and are about to find your special place. It begins to come into view as you approach. This might be a real place you have visited in the past or a place you build in your mind. It might be outdoors or inside, large or small. This is a place that is inviting, safe, and tranquil.

Allow all the details of your special place to be revealed as you explore your new surroundings.

Look around and notice all you see.

Notice everything you hear.

Notice how it feels. Is it warm or cool? Humid or dry? Is there a cozy blanket or sweater you might want to wrap yourself up in?

Notice how it smells. What scents are in the air?

Enjoy how calming it is to be here. Spend as much time as you would like, knowing you can return again.

When you are ready, say farewell to this lovely place, and make your way back to the grassy path. Although the image of your special place fades as you leave, it remains in your heart, and you can carry the calmness you feel into the rest of your day.

Return fully to your body in the present moment and grab a pen or a pencil to record your impressions. Write a full description of your special place in as much detail as possible. Remember to include how it looked, sounded, smelled, and felt.

My special place:

_____

_____

_____

_____

_____

_____

_____

_____

_____

Reflections

How was it to visit your special place? Did it come into view easily, or was it challenging to allow your creativity to freely flow?

_____

_____

_____

_____

As we age, many of us quiet the creative part of our brain and put pressure on ourselves to be serious. But our imagination is part of our wholeness, and when we welcome it back into our existence, it can provide us with access to insights and healing. That said, if the visualization exercise felt daunting or frustrating, you might decide to try it again in the future, or you might decide it isn't appealing to you. Your call entirely.

If you are open to utilizing this "Special Place" visualization as a comfort technique, I encourage you to (1) document as many specifics about your special place as possible, (2) draft an updated, personalized version of the script with all the details you listed, and (3) try it out once more. Finally, assess if any further modifications are needed. These additional steps will help ensure your script will be most effective. You can consider making an audio recording of you or someone else reading the final version if that feels useful to you.

The Benefits of Relaxation Techniques

During times of overwhelm, anxiety, pain, or sleeplessness, people can reach for a relaxation script to promote relief. This can settle everyone's nerves, providing a chance to reset. What's more, for people who have mobility limitations, but are cognitively able, a visualization can provide a sense of liberation. Some terminal conditions affect the body while leaving the mind intact. This can lead to increasing dependency, boredom, frustration, loneliness, and isolation. Traveling to a place of serenity can provide a change of scenery and mental respite.

Some people decide to incorporate these types of exercise into their time of active dying—the vigil—as it provides caregivers and visitors with a means to provide support even when reciprocal conversation is no longer possible. You might consider building this into your end-of-life wishes when we cover them more specifically later in the workbook.

Part IV

Processing: Exploring What Feels Unfinished and Undiscovered

As we make our way through life, we filter experiences through our distinctive lens, which forms from societal and familial messaging as well as our developed knowledge. Stephen R. Covey, author of *The Seven Habits of Highly Effective People*, states we all have numerous "maps" in our heads, which can be divided into two main categories. The first category includes maps of the way things are—realities— while the second includes maps of the way we think things "should" be, reflecting our values. Covey (2004, 24) believes that "we seldom question their accuracy; we're usually even unaware that we have them. We simply assume that the way we see things is the way they really are or the way they should be." The way we see things, whether based in reality or pure subjectivity, shapes our thoughts and actions.

Introspection—the examination or observation of our own mental and emotional processes—is an undeniable part of growth. When we take time to thoughtfully consider and incorporate what we are experiencing, we can then figure out who we are and how we want to *be* in the world. Otherwise, we risk operating on autopilot, moving through our days while remaining largely unaware. We'll still react to what enters or passes through our personal space, yet these reactions will be automatic, not deliberate.

When we can break free from mindlessly reacting, we can, instead, respond with intention. We can question and interpret situations more objectively, allowing us to stay in alignment with our ideals and to then embody them. The Buddhist teacher and writer Pema Chödrön (2003, 29) wrote, "The most fundamental aggression to ourselves, the most fundamental harm we can do to ourselves, is to remain ignorant by not having the courage and the respect to look at ourselves honestly and gently."

As death journalers, we are going to venture further inward during this part of our expedition, mirroring the transition we often see during people's final days and hours, when the outer world holds one's attention less and less. First, we'll delve into the topics of regret, forgiveness, and unburdening. Then, after processing specific difficulties, we will take a long look back on the lives we have lived and record the parts we wish to memorialize.

CHAPTER 7

Processing the Past

One major aspect of processing is *storying*, or the act of creating a narrative to explain past experiences. Researcher Yael Schenker and colleagues (2015) state, "Stories help us deal with surprises and upsets, make meaning out of chaos, clarify values, and build connections between past and future." We understand ourselves and the world around us better by storying our experiences.

As a doula (or simply a compassionate listener), I have observed the power of storytelling firsthand. People hold tender memories just below the surface. It's as though they are aching to share them, if only given the chance. When you quiet yourself and invite someone to go beyond small talk, they're often able to pull together commentary that gets to the core of who they are and what they believe about life.

Do you have a person in your circles available to hear about your life chronicles? Not all of us do. Even when we have people to converse with, not all listeners are adept at holding silence long enough to allow for the time and space needed to process experiences fully. An alternative or complementary option is journaling, especially when trying to resolve past anguish that might plague your memories. And working through the more difficult episodes of your life is an important first step before reviewing it fully.

Expressive Writing

Social psychologist James W. Pennebaker is best known for his studies on the therapeutic benefits of expressive writing. Pennebaker and countless researchers who have emulated his work contend that journaling for a short span can be cathartic for people who have residual effects from stressful or traumatic experiences. Pennebaker (2021) explains that part of the reason we ruminate over difficult times is that our memories remain disjointed until we work to link everything together. When we feel embarrassment or deep hurt, we don't often share it with others for fear of judgment or increased shame. This leaves our brain struggling to reconcile incidents accordingly, so our thoughts continuously swirl, which can damage our physical and mental health.

Pennebaker says when a person organizes events by putting them into words on paper, a cascade of change begins. First, there is an acknowledgment that an upsetting experience happened. As part of this validation, the writer labels what they faced and any outcomes. By structuring thoughts in this way, the person can make connections regarding consequential impacts. Pennebaker affirms this can *still the mind* as well as lead to improvements in one's social life (more talking and laughing) and health (improved sleep, focus, and immune function; less use of numbing devices). Pennebaker's research also suggests that to gain the most benefit from writing about life's traumas, writers ought to acknowledge the negative and also celebrate anything positive that occurred in the aftermath, such as personal growth and any new realizations.

The goal of expressive writing is to better understand experiences, including any losses you have endured, by being brutally honest with yourself. This writing isn't meant to be shared. You can write in whatever way is most effective for you—by hand, on a computer, or even "finger writing" in the air. To start, you can try Pennebaker's standard approach of writing for fifteen to twenty minutes for three to four days, or you can modify it. If you try it and feel better after only one day, stop there. If you feel overwhelmed after starting, then stop and lean on the healthy coping techniques you identified previously and consider professional counseling as a potential option as well.

Trying It for Yourself

If it feels appropriate to do so, try out expressive writing for yourself to see if it helps you release any heaviness you might be carrying. If there is a troubling episode haunting you, begin there. If there is more than one from your past, focus on each separately. Over the next three to four days, take fifteen to twenty minutes a day to journal about your deepest emotions and thoughts related to each experience. Write in a slow, deliberate way, allowing for the full expression of unfiltered thoughts.

Really let go and explore whatever comes to mind. You might tie memories to your childhood, important milestones, people you have loved or love now, or even your career. Consider how the experience might relate to who you have been in the past, who you are now, or who you would like to become.

Handwrite your entries on loose paper rather than within this workbook so you can relish the pure freedom of privacy. Tuck them someplace safe, as we will use them for a ritual ceremony in an upcoming exercise. After completing a round of expressive writing, add your reflections in the next entry.

Please note: There are not many reasons to avoid this activity; however, findings in a study on the topic suggest expressive writing may be contraindicated for individuals who do not typically express emotions (Niles et al. 2014). If sharing your thoughts and feelings feels uncomfortable or unsafe, please don't force yourself to journal. Make sure to assess your own style and willingness honestly before engaging.

How was the process of journaling about distressing times? Was it heavy? Did you feel lighter after expressing your memories? Take a little while to explore your experience.

While writing expressively about past challenges, I discovered:

_____

_____

_____

Upon reflection, I have realized:

_____

_____

_____

Moving forward, I will:

_____

_____

_____

Carrying unhealed trauma can be detrimental to your well-being, yet processing hardship isn't easy. Finding resolution is an undertaking. Please make sure to take good care of yourself by practicing self-compassion and seeking support when needed.

The Release

If you chose to partake in expressive writing, you now have pages of personal history that aren't meant for anyone else's eyes. You might want to read over what you divulged, or you might not. When you reach *your* place of completion with this process, it is time to let it all go. Before the release, let's discuss the restorative power of ritual in detail.

Reverent Rituals

We've heard about rituals a number of times throughout the book, including the blessing stone ritual to mark beginnings and endings and ritualistic rites of passage. Many of us are familiar with rituals in a religious sense, from the customary practices of ancient worshippers to the traditions that are commonplace in today's churches, temples, mosques, synagogues, etc. You might also be familiar with it in a more colloquial sense—the ceremonial acts we use to start our days (such as personal care tasks done in a certain order) or a regimented series of actions we use to wind down before bed at night. Ultimately, a ritual is a series of steps regularly repeated to achieve a specific end or a series of steps specially formulated to mark a special occasion.

Applied social psychologist, Jamie Gruman (2021) says rituals can offer numerous psychological advantages, such as helping us savor experiences, giving us a sense of control, and reducing anxiety. Some rituals are simple, like preparing a hot cup of coffee the same way each morning. Others require more planning, like a commitment ceremony between life partners. Some fall somewhere in between, like a solstice or full moon celebration.

Prerituals, or rituals done in advance of significant events, can heighten or enhance an occasion. An example could be following specific steps to gear yourself up for public speaking or a mindful pause before entering a person's space who is ill. And post-rituals—those performed after an event—can foster closure. In terms of death, these could include the washing and anointing of the deceased, as well as planned funerals, celebrations of life, or memorials.

As you reflect on your own life, have you developed rituals, knowingly or unknowingly? If so, what purpose do they serve? Are they formal or informal? Planned or spontaneous? As the research suggests, do they help you savor experiences, give you a sense of control, or reduce your anxiety?

_____

_____

_____

_____

Might you be interested in exploring the practice of ritual with more intention now? Following are some components to ponder as you think about how you might incorporate ritual into your days, years, and also—thinking ahead—your final phase of life.

Elements of Ritual

Some ceremonial rituals happen in response to a pressing need of the moment. They are more organic and unplanned. Others are more structured and organized. Here are four preparatory elements to keep in mind in either case. You might feel called to begin gathering ideas now for a particular event, or you might decide to return to these tips in the future. (You can download this activity from http://www.newharbinger.com/51369.)

1. Setting

Where might this ritual take place? Indoors or outside? In a familiar spot or an unusual destination?

2. Scene

Continue to build out the details. What else would be needed? What features or furniture? What time of year and day works best or would be most ideal (keeping in mind we aren't always able to control what will happen)? Who would you want to be present? What roles need to be filled? How can distractions be minimized?

3. Script

More formal rituals tend to have precise scripts, while informal ones might have a loose outline. It's often helpful for one person to take the lead, but that doesn't necessarily mean they have to do all the speaking. Rather, their role might be to officially start the ceremony and manage the overall agenda, letting others know when it is time for certain segments.

4. Sacredness

Determining what is sacred means exploring profundity. What will add meaning? What will make it memorable and special? What tone would you like your ritual to have? Light and silly or earnest and solemn? A ritual enables us to elevate what matters most in ways that resonate personally.

Integration Practice: Ritual Planning

Now you'll practice a ritual to release your expressive writing. You can begin by holding the pages of your writing in your hands, pausing to absorb all you have learned about yourself, and then conveying admiration for your resilience as well as gratitude for any support you have received.

Some people incorporate nature elements into their ceremony, such as by lighting a candle or making a fire outdoors. You can burn your writing in the fire while repeating an affirming statement like, "I release all I no longer need to hold. I carry all that serves me well." Or, if a fire doesn't appeal or isn't possible, you might tear up the pieces of paper and bury them in the earth.

Take a few minutes to dream up a modest ritual that you'll use for releasing your expressive writing and plan it out in the following space. If you chose not to participate in the expressive writing exercise, you can still participate in this ritual. You might think of a belief you hold about yourself that you're ready to let go of (for example "I'm not able to trust myself to make important decisions") and write it down on a slip of paper.

As you build out the details of your ceremony, refer to the previous section on ritual elements for inspiration. Try to avoid overly complicated steps or attaching too many expectations as to how it might go. Rigidity is antithetical to reverence. Draft a relaxed agenda with ample space for the unanticipated.

My ceremonial ritual

1. Setting

_____

_____

_____

2. Scene

_____

_____

_____

3. Script

_____

_____

_____

4. Sacredness

_____

_____

_____

Actualization

Now it is time to put your plan into action. Hold your ceremonial ritual and release your writing. After you finish, reflect on how it went and make some notes for alterations within the previous exercise or in the space below for next time. This will be a work in progress.

_____

_____

No ritual will go exactly as envisioned. There are many variables involved; we won't be able to control all aspects. If we cling too tightly to specifics, we'll lose our ability to really immerse ourselves in the process. Expect the unexpected and include generous margins. Sometimes, interruptions to the agenda can even add unforeseen value to the experience.

Final Thoughts

Marking occasions with rituals is an act of reclamation. You're saying, "This _is_ happening, and I am leaning into it." You are acknowledging a transition. Rather than minimizing its impact, you are embracing the current reality. If you stay open to this practice, it's one that can serve you through all of life's seasons. Continue to imagine how you might incorporate rituals into significant moments, for your sake and for the well-being of your loved ones.

As you did your journaling and introspective work in this chapter, thoughts about past sorrows or disappointments likely surfaced as well as things that feel undone or unsaid. Next, we'll look at ways you can continue to deal with those challenges and how to hopefully release any residual heaviness.

CHAPTER 8

Resolution Through Releasing

At the end of life, issues of regret, shame, and forgiveness come up regularly. It is not uncommon for stifled memories to return. Combing through the past seems to be critical, pressing work for people nearing the end of their days. Tenzin Kiyosaki, author and hospice chaplain, summarizes three main regrets she has heard repeatedly at the bedside (Pawlowski 2021).

1. I did not live my life of dreams.

2. I did not share my love.

3. I did not forgive.

While it is possible to seek resolution when you're terminally ill, Kiyosaki implores people to consider assessing any regrets while in good health, if and when that's possible.

Whatever your situation is at this point in time, this will be your work in this chapter. Ponder these opening questions to get started: *What dreams, big or small, have you been hoping to achieve? How guarded have you been with sharing your heart? What pains you from past relationships? Can you open yourself to resolution?*

_____

_____

_____

_____

_____

Unburdening

Suffering is an unavoidable part of the human condition. As individuals, we each face a distinct set of trials throughout our stint on Earth. As we delve into this sensitive work of returning to the past, prior injuries or injustices to our bodies, minds, and souls might return to our thoughts. Please care for yourself gently and know you don't need to uncover any times that feel too painful to revisit.

A special note on trauma: When someone has experienced trauma, there is no need to excuse a perpetrator's behavior or to "look on the bright side" in order to heal. Where there are deep wounds, there can exist an array of emotions, including rage, frustration, or sadness. If it feels safe and appropriate to extend forgiveness for a transgression or mistreatment, this can provide potential relief. If this does not feel right, forcing forgiveness can cause additional suffering. Psychotherapist Anastasia Pollock (2016) promotes an alternative, *unburdening*, which means "letting go of the power the trauma has over a person" as well as "expressing and releasing anger and other strong emotions about what happened without criticism or expectation of what needs to come next." This reframe can allow a survivor to direct their own recovery journey without undue pressure. That's how we'll approach the matter of coming to terms with and releasing the past.

Keeping with the theme of unburdening, you will now unearth any unspoken messages for others you may be holding onto. You are going to focus on words gone unshared because the associated dynamics or situations at the time felt too complicated. You can direct them to someone who is alive or deceased. These aren't messages you will necessarily share with anyone, so you can feel free to write whatever comes to mind.

As always, you direct your death wellness practices. Be sure to respect your intuition and current capacity. If the topic or timing of this exercise does not feel appropriate, you can continue to the next section. You can also reach out to trusted loved ones or clinicians or mental health professionals when needed—if, say, the exercise brings up strong feelings or memories that you need support working through.

Even though these exercises are introspective, they don't need to be done in isolation.

Letters to Others

To begin, take some time to think of a few individuals who are connected to challenging times in your life. These may be individuals who are well-known to you or people you don't know as well who've nonetheless had quite an impact on your life. For each of these people, draft a handwritten letter on a piece of paper, with the express purpose of releasing yourself from emotional heaviness.

Write as much or as little as you like. There is no right or wrong way to complete this exercise; write the letter that makes sense to you and feels beneficial. Rather than concentrating solely on what you wish could have happened differently in the past, you can also acknowledge what you may have learned or how you may have grown from hardship and heartache, as these are your takeaways to claim.

Ritual for Release

Upon completion of your letters to others, return to the ritual you planned for your expressive writing (or old belief) and again release your writing ceremoniously. Repeat a mantra focused on cleansing and liberating yourself from the hurt related to difficult events.

Afterward, you might want to pause, reflect, and journal as a way to access more clarity.

What was this experience like for you?

_____

_____

_____

_____

_____

_____

_____

Healing takes time and effort. This is one step of many in your journey. There are no miracle cures or fast tracks. You can return to this practice of unburdening when older hurts reappear or when new ones occur.

A Letter to Yourself

Now that you have finished drafting letters to others, let's turn back inward. When we recall the past, hindsight can lead us to forget we didn't have all the information beforehand. We couldn't know how everything would turn out. Take some time to pen a letter to yourself—one of self-forgiveness and gratitude—with the intention of unburdening heaviness or guilt you still might be carrying. Use a compassionate voice as though you are directing these words to a cherished friend or family member.

Dear Me,

_____

_____

_____

_____

_____

_____

_____

_____

_____

_____

_____

_____

_____

_____

_____

Reflections

You might feel drained or energized as a result of this profound work, or you might find yourself vacillating between the two. This is to be expected. Allow yourself plenty of rest and respite.

You might also feel motivated by the prior exercises to have conversations while you still can and disclose what you've been silently carrying. If so, keep in mind that not everyone will arrive at this place of readiness simultaneously. When approaching invitations to talk, you might say something along the lines of, "I've been doing more thinking about the past lately. I know what's done is done, but I'd like the chance to talk about what happened and how it affected our relationship if you're willing—for the sake of reconciliation."

Some of the people you ask will be willing to have these conversations. Even if the other person resists, though, you still have the option of drafting letters—which you might send or might not. Either way, the writing can lighten your emotional burden.

The overarching aim so far in this section has been to strengthen connections within yourself and to your stories to foster clarity and harmony. If, after exhuming past adversities, your thoughts feel noisy and unrelenting, consider utilizing this meditative exercise as a way to recenter.

Visualization Exercise: Blue Sky

Settle yourself into your space and body, slow your breathing, and then read the following imagery.

Imagine the sun in a clear, blue sky—radiant, life-giving, and warm. Now, see clouds moving in on a cold wind, covering the sky in a gray blanket. Above the clouds, the sun continues shining, unconditionally, indifferent to the presence of clouds. Above the cloud cover, the sky is still blue. Notice how you feel when you think of the dark clouds. Now notice how you feel when you think of the light of the sun shining high above it all.

(This exercise was adapted from "Mindfulness for Prolonged Grief" by from Kumar et al. 2013.)

Afterthoughts

When submerged in darkness, it's easy to forget that the sun is always shining, even when hidden behind clouds. The "Blue Sky Visualization" can be an uplifting reminder during a cloudy spell.

You might choose to utilize this exercise by envisioning the sky as your essential self, always steady and present while thoughts and feelings are clouds that change shape, dissipate, and float by. Everything passes—sensations, interactions, acute periods of grief and sadness, and even lifetimes. Acknowledging transience can help you weather the suffering caused by adversity—and perhaps even transcend it.

CHAPTER 9

Your Life Review

As you live your life, you not only experience a variety of phases, but you also pass through different developmental stages. Clinicians and researchers attempt to categorize and define these stages based on social and psychological patterns within the average human growth trajectory. These stages don't necessarily start and end at the same point for each person, nor do they always contain the exact same components. But there are many notable commonalities people share.

Reviewing developmental theories can shed light onto what you're facing, fearing, and hoping for as you age, and perhaps make us all feel a little less alone in our humanness.

Psychoanalyst Erik Erikson (1950), who is best known for his stage theory of psychosocial development, argues that people construct their sense of self over the entirety of the lifespan. Erikson outlines eight key stages in human development. Each comes with a central conflict and offers potential positive outcomes to be carried forward—and the stages build upon each other. The first five begin at infancy and extend through adolescence.

Stage 1: Trust versus mistrust

Positive outcomes: safety and security, and the virtue of hope

Stage 2: Autonomy versus shame and doubt

Positive outcomes: self-sufficiency and independence, and the virtue of will

Stage 3: Initiative versus guilt

Positive outcomes: self-efficacy and the virtue of purpose

Stage 4: Industry versus inferiority

Positive outcomes: confidence and the virtue of competence

Stage 5: Identity versus confusion

Positive outcomes: an integrated and cohesive sense of self and the virtue of fidelity

Stage 6: Intimacy versus isolation

This stage spans from the end of adolescence until middle adulthood. The challenge of this stage is to build loving, lasting relationships with others, leading to feelings of connectedness and belonging, and the virtue of love.

The final two stages help explain our tendencies in middle and older adulthood—and, it seems, as we struggle with mortality at any age. Since they're more applicable to death wellness, let's go into detail about each one.

Stage 7: Generativity versus stagnation

During middle adulthood, people often become more focused on contributing something to society and making their mark on the world. Activities that reinforce generativity include caregiving, volunteering, mentoring, and finding success in a meaningful career.

On the flipside of generativity is stagnation, which points to a lack of substantive involvement in life. This leads to decreased feelings of satisfaction and potentially a "midlife crisis." Or, for those who are terminally ill at any age, stagnation can lead to an experience of languishing.

The key virtue of this stage—when we're able to reinforce generativity and resist or work through stagnation—is "care," which involves tending to loved ones and colleagues as well as to one's community and future generations. This reinforces the pattern of focusing on relationships more so than materialistic concerns during the end of life.

Stage 8: Integrity versus despair

The final stage of psychosocial development takes place in late adulthood and involves looking back over one's life. When we reflect and feel fulfilled, we are able to develop a sense of integrity and coherence—a sense our life is complete and that it mattered. Indications of integrity include acceptance, a sense of wholeness and success, and feeling at peace. When we have regrets, on the other hand, we may experience resentment or despair over a life we see as "misspent." We might ruminate over mistakes and feel depressed, aimless, or hopeless. In the end, the key virtue of this stage is "wisdom," which bolsters a sense of closure and completeness, which can lessen the fear of death.

While each of Erikson's stages presents as distinct, in reality, life is much more fluid. It's not the case that those who achieve resolution within these psychosocial conflicts are continuously basking in generativity and ego integrity. Instead, people inevitably find themselves at different points along the spectrum depending on their current circumstance and internal reserves. Ultimately, healthy personal growth involves regularly rebalancing and recalibrating as we vacillate between states.

Erikson's life stage theory reinforces the value of symbolic immortality efforts, namely projecting ourselves into the future. Again, your life mission does not need to be grandiose to count. Most of us build our legacy out of quiet endeavors, small acts of kindness, and the connections we forge with those around us.

Where do you find yourself along these developmental stages? Where have you been in the past? Where do you aspire to end up? What aspects of the stages speak to you at this present moment?

_____

_____

_____

_____

_____

_____

_____

Life Review

With your evolving development in mind, your next activity is drafting a life review—a document that captures the events and experiences of your existence thus far. You have a choice as to how much of your past you'd like to write about in the following pages.

You might decide to start on scrap paper, documenting an unfiltered, honest account of your life's highs and lows. In this way—similar to the expressive writing exercise—it might be appealing to freewrite without worrying if anyone else will read it. You'll be writing to yourself, for your own personal growth. As a second step (or as your first step if you decide to bypass freewriting), you can draft a life review that feels appropriate to share with others—either typed, on paper, or within the blank section at the end of this chapter. There, you can include selective portions of your life story—the parts you might want others to know about.

Sharing your personal history is a generous act. By doing so, you are passing down lessons learned, and preserving a way of life that might otherwise go unknown. As researcher Sherry Hamby (2013) says, "People who have found their voice, shared their story, and reaffirmed their values often find a sense of peace and a hopefulness that they did not have before."

Further, by revealing your reflections to loved ones, you can use your own journey as a means to support them on theirs. This is not to say everyone who hears your life story will necessarily walk the same path, but inevitably, there will be rich learning available. The established relationships you have with some of the people who'll read your story—perhaps children, relatives, friends, and others—will be strengthened, and new ones that extend across generations may be forged. And there are benefits to reap in drafting a life review even if you don't plan to leave your story or this workbook to others. As Hamby explains, "Emotional, autobiographical storytelling can be a path to truly owning your story."

How to Begin

Whether you decide to (a) write an unfiltered life record on scrap paper and then add only choice highlights in the following section, (b) contemplate a comprehensive life review in your mind and then write out the portions you would like to share, or (c) focus solely on the parts of the past you would like to feature, you can decide to organize your life review by either decades or subjective eras.

- Decades: Starting with your early childhood, reflect on each decade of your life.

- Eras: Divide your life into different episodes, for instance, childhood, school years, early adulthood, specific jobs you held, relationships, post-retirement, grandparenthood, and the like.

To recall what happened, you can also ask yourself the *who, what, when, where, why,* and *how* questions that follow. These are merely to help you gather ideas as you recall aspects of your life during each decade or era. Feel free to explore other topics that arise naturally when you start writing your actual review. You'll see there's space for your full life story after these initial questions. (You can download this activity at http://www.newharbinger.com/51369.)

Who?

Who were you in terms of your roles and personality? Who did you spend your time with? Who were you close to? Whom did you love?

_____

_____

_____

What?

What was important during this period? What were the most memorable moments? What were your favorite pastimes, interests, shops, or restaurants? What did you believe back then?

_____

_____

_____

When?

When were there turning points? When did significant change happen?

_____

_____

_____

Where?

Where did you live? Where did you spend your days? Where did you travel to or visit?

_____

_____

_____

Why?

Why do these certain memories, activities, and connections stand out to you?

_____

_____

_____

How?

How do you feel about this time period, upon reflection? How did you deal with any hardship or heartache? How did this time shape the person you are today?

_____

_____

_____

Writing Your Life Story

Drafting personal chronicles reinforces one's sense of identity, which is valuable anytime during adulthood, but is especially crucial during times of illness. As a doula, I often remind my clients: *You are not your health status—you are still you.* Whatever your physical condition is currently and however many years you've lived so far, utilize the next several pages to document what you'd like to record of your history.

May this be a restoration of your wholeness.

My History

Hopefully your life review can become a source of strength in the days to come, as you revisit it, reflect on it, and continue to add to it. And hopefully the process of sorting through your past for pivotal moments has proven illuminating.

Part V

Projects: Clarifying and Sharing Your Authentic Self

As you recalled the past while drafting your life review, you were—of course—featured as the primary character. You provided the lens, voice, and substance for each story. Who was that *you* though? Were you the same person the whole way through? Were you different versions of yourself or rather an evolution of the *you* you're destined to become? Take a moment to consider these questions and write about them if you'd like.

_____

_____

_____

_____

_____

As stated in the beginning of the workbook, we need to first determine who we are before we can share ourselves with others or provide specific instructions for our preferred care. In this section, you'll continue to mull over intrapersonal themes as you further define yourself—internally, relationally, and behaviorally. Additionally, you can explore whether all the aspects of yourself are in alignment by contemplating: *Is there congruence between who I feel I am, who I say I am, how others perceive me, and how I act?*

As you work through the projects in this section, you will not only be uncovering who you are, but you will also discern what you might need from those who want to understand and honor your true wishes. When all these elements are in place, alongside complementary layers of compassionate medical support, you can better access unified, personalized care.

CHAPTER 10

Your Core Self

Core self is your true self or most authentic self. According to psychotherapist Rachel Eddins, it is your "inner wisdom, inner nurturer, wise self, feeling self, or inner voice" (Tartakovsky 2016). How often do you tune in to your most authentic self? How frequently do you listen to your inner wisdom?

_____

_____

Most of the time, we operate at a surface level: *I'm hungry. I'm tired. I'm fine.* However, when we delve deeper, we find more nuanced layers. One person might uncover a quiet yearning for connection, while another might realize they enjoy feelings of contentment associated with healthy choices they're making. Someone else might detect a listlessness related to a lack of purpose. What's simmering underneath your exterior?

Working through these layers to discover your core self is a valuable practice. It can help reveal your personality traits and solidify your values. This exploration also helps to keep priorities top of mind to inspire meaningful living.

Favorites

A broad and simple starting place is with our *favorites*, or what we really like, as they highlight much about us—our interests and preferences in addition to what entertains and moves us. This is a great entry point for accessing your core self.

Years ago, I incorporated this technique into the support I offered a young father through his end-of-life journey. He worried his children would not remember him as they grew up. This devastating thought loomed over his final months. It had prompted him to get an admirable head start on legacy work, with his partner's help, before he and I worked together. Still, we continued to capture all we could about who he was and what he'd accomplished.

His illness progressed, drastically affecting cognition. He could no longer recount special moments or verbalize future messages as his energy waned and ability to communicate worsened. So, we resorted to more simple questions that required one-word answers—a favorites list. I focused on what I knew to be meaningful topics, like sports teams and musical artists, while sprinkling in others to round it out.

I have no doubt his children will treasure the gifts he created. When they revisit them, they will be able to know their father even better. And with his favorites list, as they develop their own hobbies and interests, they can compare and contrast theirs with what he had highlighted. I can envision them cheering for their father's favorite sports team, and I can see them reaching the age when they can watch their father's favorite movie, feeling close to him once more.

Take some time to complete your own favorites list in the following exercise. Leave any sections blank that do not beckon an answer. Also, leave more than one answer, if you'd like. And feel free to add more topics within the blank fields.

My favorite:

Song _____

Book _____

Movie _____

TV show _____

Food _____

Restaurant _____

Place on earth _____

Vacation _____

Color _____

Activity (sport or hobby) _____

Season _____

Weather _____

Holiday _____

Animal/pet _____

Person/people _____

_____

_____

_____

_____

In my own death journal, my primary concern has been to pass along tidbits about myself and life history to my loved ones so they can have continued access to me, even in my absence. I hope they'll sense my essence on each page.

One of my ongoing entries has been my "Happiness Is" list. When I revisit this particular section, I see evidence of numerous additions. There are different inks, and my handwriting varies as well. Some of the initial entries are large as though I never imagined filling the entire page. More recent adds are smaller, squeezed in next to others as space is now quite limited.

My main goal is to share with my beloveds what makes my heart beam in hopes that when reading it, they might smile in response.

Happiness Is...

As you begin this reflective exercise, first ask yourself: *What does happiness mean to me? What does it feel like? Is it deep satisfaction? Uplifting joy? Is it a blend of many sensations?*

_____

_____

_____

_____

And now, however you have defined happiness, allow yourself a stroll down memory lane to recall as many moments of it as possible. Where do you find yourself in these memories associated with pure happiness? Are you dancing to live music? Is there a purring cat snuggling in your lap? Is happiness a big bowl of salad with homegrown vegetables? Is it skiing in fresh powder, swimming in a clear lake, or some other kind of physical activity? Is happiness time spent with certain friends or family members? Is it time spent alone?

Use the following page to write your list of happiness sources. Your entries can be brief or lengthy or a combination of the two.

Happiness is...

_____

_____

_____

_____

_____

_____

_____

_____

_____

_____

_____

_____

_____

_____

Reflections

Are you smiling or chuckling as you reminisce about happy times? Are your eyes welling up with tears? Are there common themes present within your list, like connection, nurturance, or quiet solitude? Are there more planned events or seemingly random ones? Have there been certain seasons of your life flush with happiness?

_____

_____

_____

_____

The answers you have written in your list will likely have positive associations with enjoyable times. Take time to relish and bask in these memories.

Contemplating happiness brings us closer to our core—to our *feeling self.* As children, we tend not to filter bliss. We express it without a second thought. As we age, we often become more reserved. Have you stopped to wonder why? Of course, not every setting will be an appropriate one to launch into a happy dance, yet are we allowing ourselves the opportunity at all? Anywhere? At any point? Can you extend an invitation to yourself to celebrate delight without reserve?

Now that you have spent time compiling happiness into list form, you might notice and welcome even more doses of joy in the days to come. You now have a heightened level of awareness. You might also find yourself seeking out opportunities that promote happiness. How might you invite and integrate enjoyment more often?

_____

_____

_____

_____

In addition to potentially impacting your everyday life, the lists you are drafting within this chapter have the potential to become useful tools for people offering you support through times of need. Even during the most difficult moments, people often appreciate the relief felt in a smile shared. Watching a much-loved movie or playing a favorite song can transform a person's mood. Caregivers and concerned loved ones can infuse glimmers of joy from these stated sources of happiness to balance out some of the intensity when times get tough.

After writing my "Happiness Is" list in my death journal, I recognized the many benefits it contained. Not only would my loved ones have a clearer sense of me, but they would also be able to care for me better. This realization led me to create a second list, with the intention of expanding upon the informative ideas I could supply.

Comfort Is...

Similar to your "Happiness Is" list, we will now focus on the topic of comfort, which moves us closer to the *inner nurturer* at our core. This is a more tender realm as it houses a range of memories, even uncomfortable ones. To travel here, we must be willing to become more vulnerable. To begin, consider these opening questions: *When you imagine yourself feeling completely comfortable, what does it look like? What does it feel like?*

_____

_____

_____

For this particular exercise, your task will be to compile a list of what brings your whole being into a place of calmness and serenity. Of course, the need to seek comfort often follows a stressful situation. So, as you recall these moments, please go easy on yourself. Past suffering or traumatic events may enter your thoughts. You can choose to explore those times, perhaps through expressive writing or shift your focus away from them, depending on what feels best.

Instead of recalling the details of a challenging time, you might decide to concentrate on how you accessed comfort. Whom or what did you seek out? Meditate on comfort—what it means and specific examples from your lifetime. Do you tend to seek comfort in nature? Or do you find it inside your own home? Do you sense comfort when interacting with people, or might you retreat into the stillness of your own mind?

What is your image of serenity? One of opening a favorite book of poetry while sitting in a favorite chair? Or is it submerging yourself in a warm bath with aromatic salts? Is there a certain fabric involved—soft flannel or smooth silk perhaps? Is there music playing in the background? Are there other sounds, like a certain person's voice or maybe ocean waves?

Your compilation won't be exactly the same as anyone else's. And there are no wrong answers. Recall your personal sources of comfort and list them in the next space.

Comfort is...

_____

_____

_____

_____

_____

_____

_____

_____

_____

_____

_____

_____

Reflections

What patterns, if any, emerged in your reflections on comfort? Have you leaned on a variety of strategies to experience comfort? Can you name a "tried and true" example—one that repeats itself?

_____

_____

_____

Has your definition of comfort changed throughout the years? Do you prefer a type of peacefulness that is quick and fleeting or something that is more lasting and meaningful? Would you consider your sources healthy or unhealthy, or perhaps a mix of both?

_____

_____

_____

Like your "Happiness Is" list, your comfort compilation can be a running list—one you expand on as time passes.

And now that comfort is on your mind, you might find yourself more attuned to it. Next time you're experiencing comfort, cue yourself to pause, breathe, and settle into it more fully. Immerse yourself. Engage all of your senses. If you're sliding warm wool socks onto your feet, revel in it. If you are held in a loving embrace, sink into it. If the warmth of sunshine soaks into your skin like good medicine, relish the sensation.

These moments do not always need to be profound to be significant—they merely need to be acknowledged and appreciated. The comforting feel of your familiar robe could be easily missed or thoroughly enjoyed. It's a matter choice—an orientation.

You might even find that as you take note of tranquility more often, any competing frustrations dissipate somewhat; that is, tranquility, when we're aware of it, can act as an antidote of sorts to frustration. And now, you have a number of ideas at the ready to utilize when facing demands and challenges.

Using Your Lists as Care Tools

If you decide to share these lists with others, they will have tools to employ. You are creating a personalized care kit of sorts. When we are ill or stressed, support is vital. Humans are interdependent beings meant to companion one another. However, knowing how to offer support can be difficult for friends and family members. Even professional care providers sometimes struggle to know what might be most beneficial for a particular patient or client.

Your lists help answer the often frustratingly broad question: *What can I do?* You are supplying others with specific ways to tend to your distress. These are hand-chosen, customized approaches, which can alleviate fear while empowering people to step up and step in.

If instead, we leave people guessing how to soothe us, they will likely employ the Golden Rule. They will offer to us what *they* would personally appreciate. This might work, but it might very well not. For example, some people seek touch—a hand held or a gentle massage. Others would rather have a kind presence close by without any physical contact. By providing instruction, people can care for you in ways you actually want. Plus, you might even have more confidence to ask for what you need now that you have identified it.

Gratitude

Reflecting on comfort and happiness can naturally lead to feelings of gratitude. According to psychiatry researchers Randy Sansone and Lori Sansone (2010), gratitude is "the appreciation of what is valuable and meaningful to oneself and represents a general state of thankfulness and/or appreciation." Thus, we can categorize gratitude as a state or a trait. As a state, gratitude is thankfulness for a kind or generous act, which is its more fleeting form. Gratitude can also be a lasting trait—a perspective through which we perceive our experiences as a matter of course.

When we pay attention to our favorite things, as well as to what brings us happiness and comfort, we tend to feel more fortunate because we are focused on goodness—what's going well in our life and how much that means to us. Many mental health clinicians encourage formal gratitude practices, like gratitude lists, and believe these interventions can enhance well-being (Lamas et al. 2014). Hence, it seems there's a positive feedback loop within these core-self practices.

For the purposes of the next exercise, review your favorites, happiness, and comfort lists to encourage a sense of gratitude. By doing so, you will again journey to the center of your core self. Reflect on your good fortune, past and present. Is there anything not yet featured within your three lists in this chapter? If so, include them in the following space provided. You may also repeat and reaffirm aforementioned entries from the other lists that are applicable.

I am grateful for...

_____

_____

_____

_____

_____

_____

_____

_____

_____

_____

_____

LIFE

Now that you have reflected on sources of happiness, comfort, and gratitude, you can begin to extend outward what resides at your core. As a way to do this, we're going to write acrostic poems featuring the word "life." For this type of poem, a certain word is spelled out vertically, and as you go downward, each letter starts a new line of the poem.

Here are two examples of an acrostic poem with the word LIFE:

Love makes

It all

Feel

Everlasting

Looking through

Internal keepsakes

Fosters gratitude and

Ethereal insights

Now it's your turn to write a LIFE poem. You can base your poem on your overarching views—perhaps featuring tenets of living well or thoughts about why we exist at all. Your poem can be inspirational advice or something more personal. It can be heartfelt, serious, or playful. It can rhyme or not. It can be long or short. You can write multiple poems if you feel called to.

Your acrostic LIFE poem(s):

L

I

F

E

L

I

F

E

Beliefs

In the previous exercise, you likely revealed some of your life philosophies. Now, we'll dive deeper into this topic and tap into our *wise self* by further exploring beliefs. Your beliefs can have roots in religion, spirituality, lived experience, or even hopeful dreams. They can be reverent in nature ("I believe that volunteerism is a virtue"), but they can also be light ("I believe in fairytales").

What are your convictions? What is unshakable despite any situation and through all challenges? What do you know to be true or what do you wish to be true?

_____

_____

_____

_____

Before adding written responses to the next exercise, first contemplate your core beliefs and their value. What do they add to your life? How do they influence your choices and path?

_____

_____

_____

_____

Make a compilation list of personal beliefs by completing the following statements.

I believe in…

_____

_____

_____

_____

I believe that…

_____

_____

_____

_____

Take time to review your stated beliefs. Did any of your statements surprise you? Did you allow yourself leeway to include a variety of answers? Are any of them positive affirmations you repeat to alter your mindset? Are they sourced from magical or wishful thinking, or are they more practical, in other words tested and proven? Allow yourself to wonder about your beliefs while suspending any judgment.

_____

_____

_____

_____

How would it feel to share this list with others? Are you open and vocal about any of these guideposts? Do you keep some private? Would you like to examine or question any in more depth? Would you like to strengthen any of them?

_____

_____

_____

_____

Our beliefs often mirror our thought patterns. As mentioned before, what we think about ourselves, others, and the world informs our framework. When we seek to gain more clarity about our viewpoints, we develop more agency over our reactions and behaviors. Thus, we can make more thoughtful, purposeful choices.

Given that, are your beliefs in alignment with who you feel you are and how you act?

_____

_____

Returning

This chapter offered numerous invitations to uncover (and remember) your truest self—who you are at your core. You began by naming your "favorites," identifying best-loved interests and preferences. Then, you examined the concepts of happiness and comfort, drafting lists that reflect what elates and calms you while illuminating your innermost wisdom. From that place of clarity, you paused to embrace gratitude and appraise your beliefs.

Often, these practices activate spiraling reverberations in our lives as we live them; they enhance our pursuit of meaning. Achieving and stabilizing our ever-shifting state of mortality awareness requires mindful effort. So, as you turn from this book back to your day-to-day life, keep questions like these in mind: *What am I allowing and inviting? What am I intentionally avoiding?*

The main task you've worked on in this chapter—the task of returning to yourself—is a lifelong practice. We are developing into ourselves until our very last breath. Now that you have allowed your inner voice to convey such genuine parts of yourself, you will focus more keenly on legacy work, including remembrance gifts specially made for others.

CHAPTER 11

Remembrance Projects

Now that you have gazed inward at your core self, it's time to survey the people around you. Who is important or special to you? What relationships and bonds are significant? Who might you want to pay tribute to as part of your death journaling efforts?

_____

_____

_____

_____

_____

Letters for Sharing

In prior exercises, you drafted letters for releasing as well as letters to yourself. Your next invitation is to write letters to friends, neighbors, relatives, coworkers, or acquaintances who have made an enduring impact. Your first decision is whether to direct one general letter to your whole community or to create individual letters. You might even complete both projects, as they can serve different purposes.

General. Some people compose a special message to be read aloud during their post-passage services or to have featured within a printed bulletin or obituary. Some like to gather their people before their death for a living funeral to share heartfelt messages in person. A general letter is appropriate for any of these options.

In it, you can include themes we have covered within the workbook already, such as happiness, gratitude, forgiveness, beliefs, your "why," and your life mantras, along with certain memories or milestones.

You might feel a sense of completion after one paragraph, or you might need many pages to express yourself. If it's appealing, take some time to jot down notes in the following space and then write a full draft in the next section.

Dearest _____ (loved ones, friends and family members, community),

_____

_____

_____

_____

_____

_____

_____

_____

_____

_____

_____

_____

Specific. If you choose to draft separate messages for chosen individuals—whether it's in addition to or instead of a group letter—you might include particular sentiments and pressing reminders that wouldn't be suitable for a broad letter. These notes can be short or lengthy. Here are some prompts, focused on relationships and legacy, that can serve as inspiration for content. (You can download this activity from http://www.newharbinger.com/51369.)

Relationship-focused:

Who you are to me…

What I respect/admire/enjoy about you…

What our relationship means to me…

The imprint you have made on my life…

What I hope you will remember…

Legacy-focused:

What matters most to me…

What has inspired me…

What shaped my perspectives…

What I have learned…

What I have struggled with…

What I have overcome…

What I accept…

Who comes to mind as you consider writing specific letters? And what do you want to remember to incorporate within these remembrance letters? Jot down initial ideas for safekeeping here.

_____

_____

_____

_____

_____

If you are planning to create personalized messages, now is the time! You can either write these by hand or type them. You can also consider recording yourself reading your letters (video or audio). Keep in mind, this is not only a writing assignment; it's an emotional experience. You will be sifting through the past as you document thoughts. And remember, customization is key, as is thoughtfulness. What will the recipients of your letters appreciate most?

Take a few days with this project, and then return to journal about it.

_____

_____

_____

_____

_____

_____

_____

Reflections

How was that to brainstorm final farewells? It can feel weighty. We want to get it *just right*. This fear can actually stop us from completing anything. Please keep in mind that mourners will want to hear from you—your distinct voice and mannerisms through your writing. Capturing these sincere messages is one way of many to share parts of yourself with those you care about.

Make sure to store any completed letters in a place where they will be found, like a top drawer of a desk, within a keepsake box, or tucked into your death journal. If you're storing them digitally, leave detailed instructions about how people can access them.

Additional Projects

In addition to letters and recordings, there are several other remembrance gifts to consider, depending on your interests and energy level. Before my Aunt Nancy died, she asked her daughter to finish prepping a future birthday present for me (a series of framed collages with cutout messages on a backdrop featuring my favorite flower) and asked my cousin to deliver them to me if she could not. I can't tell you how much solace that last display of love gave me, after two months of missing my aunt's physical presence, and how much it warmed my heart to know even death couldn't break our bond. I have heard countless grievers yearn for such a gift.

What projects call to you? Perhaps a memory garden, death journal, cookbook, or other handmade craft? Some of these can be started, or even completed, alongside loved ones while you are alive—promoting togetherness—while others might feel better suited as legacy gifts to be given after your death.

Memory gardens. When my cousin's mother-in-law died, I gave her two bleeding heart plants along with my condolences. With help from her young kids, they made a special "Nana Garden" to memorialize her life. Spaces like these can become a place to visit when seeking a sense of connection to someone who has died as well as a chance to witness the seasons and life cycle.

Some people add a bench to their memory garden for quiet sits as well as décor, like lighting and chimes. Even if the family leaves the property at some point, they might be able to dig up some perennials for their next home. If not, they leave knowing a part of their person's essence can continue on in the form of beauty and blossoms. I often call my outdoor flower areas "collector's gardens" because I have plants (divided perennials) from my great-grandmother, grandmother, my aunt-in-law and her grandmother, and also countless neighbors and friends. They each tell a story of kinship and legacy.

Death journals. Similar to my death journal that I have described—a scrapbook in which I store notes, quotes, poetry, song lyrics, mementos, and instructions for my care—you can create your own assortment of offerings. Some version of this workbook could work well. Or you could do something different. You might make one death journal for all your loved ones (with general or individual messages contained within it), or you might make a number of smaller keepsakes for different people—each with its own unique flair that honors the relationship you share.

Cookbooks. Many of us demonstrate care to others through cooking. Whether it's a favorite birthday cake or a hearty casserole, the thought and energy we put into making a special treat or meal often feels like love manifested. Many treasured holidays and traditions showcase certain menu items.

Do you enjoy cooking or baking? If so, think about your personal specialties. What are you known for in terms of your culinary skills? What do your loved ones regularly request? Some recipes have been passed down from generation to generation, while others might be all your own. You can capture them within a legacy cookbook. Sprinkle in generous helpings of memories associated with the meals and "pro tips" for those who will receive it.

Handmade and heartfelt gifts. Are you a quilter or do you know someone skilled in sewing who might want to assist you with a project? Some people turn a person's collection of souvenir T-shirts into a patchwork quilt. Others might incorporate signature clothing items, like a comfy bathrobe, favorite sweater, and lap blanket, into a special keepsake like a "bereavement bear" (a stuffed bear made with chosen fabrics). I commissioned a friend to turn one of my deceased grandfather's flannel shirts into a pillow for my grandmother so she could squeeze it when her arms felt empty.

You might also consider plaster molds—perhaps of your hand holding a beloved's or a fingerprint mold that might be worn as jewelry. "Thought rocks" can be a nice, simple activity as well. Collect rocks that have a somewhat flat surface and paint or write messages of affection or inspiration on them, either for someone in particular or loved ones in general.

Take a few minutes to ponder these projects and any others that might come to mind. What appeals? What doesn't? Would you want to work on any of these now or soon, or would you prefer to leave requests for efforts to happen after your death?

_____

_____

_____

_____

_____

_____

Bequeathing

In addition to creating gifts, consider what you already have at your disposal that you might offer to others. First, think through these opening questions: _What do your belongings mean to you? Do you have a collection of art? Stamps? Coins? Albums? Have ancestors passed down family heirlooms to you? Do you have_ *cherished jewelry? Pieces of furniture? Dish sets? What are your most prized possessions? What might you want to gift to someone now or after your time of dying?*

_____

_____

_____

_____

Now consider how you might want to disperse these treasures. It's helpful to note that some families are able to divvy up the personal effects of a deceased loved one equitably, allowing the process to become grounds for connection and healing. For others, misdirected grief can incite turmoil, leading to arguments and fractures in the family system.

How might your loved ones deal with all that's left behind in the aftermath of your departure? How clearly will you need to spell out your wishes?

_____

_____

_____

Note, we're narrowing in on physical assets here, rather than money bequests or your entire estate or the disposition of more ephemeral assets, like access to online accounts. For more guidance on these sorts of completion tasks, visit the appendices for a helpful reminder list.

In terms of gifting your physical goods, you will need to complete legal forms outside of this workbook to make any wishes official. But as a precursor to designating the beneficiaries of your "tangible personal property" in a will—or reviewing and updating your current will to ensure accurateness—take some time to now evaluate and eliminate what you no longer need and what no longer serves you.

Death Decluttering

Death decluttering, or sorting through what you've accumulated, is *memento mori* in action. It means remembering you are mortal and committing to doing constructive work in advance of life's final stage. Death decluttering is also a cathartic way to practice accepting impermanence. It's more than a spring cleaning—it involves a thorough assessment of what you own to see what you can release now to save others the daunting task later.

There are a number of potential benefits associated with the practice of death decluttering. Purging unnecessary or extraneous possessions can help:

- Create order. When our spaces aren't organized, we often feel scatter-brained. Sorting and prioritizing can sharpen our focus so we can spend time in more meaningful ways.

- Lower anxiety and stress. An orderly home can calm our minds and aid in relaxation.

- Lead to a sense of pride in what we've accomplished and relief that someone else won't have to tackle as much on our behalf.

Tips

To set yourself up for this challenge, follow these suggestions:

1. Start with belongings that have less emotional charge, and then work your way toward special relics and souvenirs.

2. Don't feel like you need to get rid of everything. We piece together our environment with things. The *feel* of your space is important. Take stock of your material collections with equal portions of honesty and self-compassion.

3. Consider spreading this task over a stretch of time. Take breaks and allow yourself moments to reminisce and even detour temporarily. The items you uncover might become inspiration for death journal entries or letters for sharing.

4. As you're sorting through your stuff, ask yourself:

   - *What emotions or memories are attached to this object?*

   - *Do I need to keep it to maintain that link, or might there be another way to honor it, such as writing about it within a journal entry or taking a photo of it for a scrapbook?*

   - *Does it bring me joy?*

- *Do I have good cause to keep it? Is it useful? Necessary? Valuable? Uplifting?*
- *Is there someone I could gift this to—now or in the future—who might need or cherish it?*

Chances are, you will unearth priceless possessions associated with key moments in your life while decluttering. But do remember: *You are not your things.* You are *you*. Your things might reflect aspects of your personhood, yet they do not define you. You exist beyond them. And with this knowledge in mind, consider: *What might you be ready to let go of?* Once you do, you'll likely experience a deepened appreciation for the items you've thoughtfully chosen to keep.

Following any death-decluttering efforts, return to journal about the experience.

_____

_____

_____

_____

_____

_____

_____

_____

Now we'll take some time to think about what you might do with the items you've decided to bequeath to others.

Bestowal Ceremonies

Passing down possessions is yet another way of sharing a part of you with others. Some people decide to gift valuable collections to an organization, gallery, or museum. Others choose a specific friend or family member to receive something they've held sacred. Sometimes, when a person knows time is short, they might hold a ceremonial disbursement while alive; for example, an artist who gathers their people together and offers each a piece of their work. One woman who had an incredible assortment of scarves invited each of her deathbed visitors to pick out their favorite one as a legacy gift before saying goodbye. I imagine many of those visitors wore their special scarf to her funerary services.

As you think about your own preferences, would you want to hold a bestowal ceremony? If so, do you feel called to create a ritual for this in advance? Would you want to plan for it to occur before your time of death or after? What might you give to whom?

_____

_____

_____

_____

_____

_____

_____

_____

As you work with the activities of this chapter, try to keep in mind that while you might have strong associations with certain belongings, other people might not feel the same (or they might not have room to add your things to their space). Saddening as it can be, this is a possibility you might have to face. Remember, your things are not *you*. They're also not your interpersonal relationships. Both are intangible and invaluable.

Part VI

Planning: Drafting Your Wishes for Care

Developing your wishes for end-of-life care means pulling from all the work you have already completed, including compassion principles, visualizations and relaxation scripts, mortality and impermanence practices, comfort and coping techniques, rituals and ceremonies, journaling, life review, and remembrance projects. You will now harvest choice elements of this bounty to construct a succinct, custom atlas for those offering you support.

As a doula who holds space at both birth and death, I have assisted with the creation of written wishes countless times, encouraging clients to consider these a communication tool that fosters person-centered care. When helping people prepare for the end of life, I often talk them through a deathbed visualization, asking them to build out the picture of the environment in their mind. You'll have an opportunity to try this yourself in an upcoming exercise.

Once, when processing the deathbed visualization, a gentleman shared that his dying space was fully decorated for his favorite holiday, Christmas. This wasn't something he had thought of previously or planned in advance. It just appeared. And it was "wonderful," he said. At that moment, he decided that whatever the time of year, if his death were imminent and it was possible, he wanted to be surrounded by the sights, sounds, and smells of Christmas.

I often share this example because I found it so delightfully surprising and inspired. Many people have a favorite holiday, season, or ambience that can be incorporated. Plus, it's pretty manageable to pack up a box of special décor and set it up almost anywhere—a home, hospital, or hospice house.

Getting specific about what you would find appealing during a time of great need is such a gift—to others and yourself. Some people prefer quiet serenity. Others want life to continue on as normally as possible around them. Of course, not everyone is sure about all the details, and it's not necessary to pretend you are clear on everything. It's actually more important to remain flexible and build adaptable plans. The unexpected is bound to occur, although it might not fully interrupt your process if your team can respond with agility and creativity, keeping what matters most top of mind.

Ultimately, throughout this final section, you will be pondering the *who, what, when, where, why,* and *how* questions to clarify your preferences. To start, though, think about any preliminary ideas you have about your deathbed space.

_____

_____

_____

_____

_____

_____

_____

_____

_____

In addition to envisioning yourself within this ideal death nest, you might also think about those around you and how they'll be experiencing your time of dying. Jennifer O'Brien, author of *The Hospice Doctor's Widow: A Journal*, mourned the loss of her husband through writing and making digital art. She graciously made this bespoke piece for this workbook, knowing you—dear reader—would be grappling with the weighty task of envisioning the end.

O'Brien describes *Precious Time* as a particular type of time:

Precious Time is when you engage fully and make your love and care known because death is likely or imminent. There is no dress rehearsal for death. We do not get do-overs. This may be one of the biggest events of a person's lifetime, and those who live on will carry it in memoriam for the rest of their days. Precious Time is when you say what you need to say and don't say what you might regret.

Surviving loved ones often lament, "I thought we had more time," or "I didn't realize so-and-so was actively dying." Identifying Precious Time as such will hopefully help people experience their death or that of a loved one with less remorse. We need to be willing to talk about end-of-life in general, but especially as it approaches.

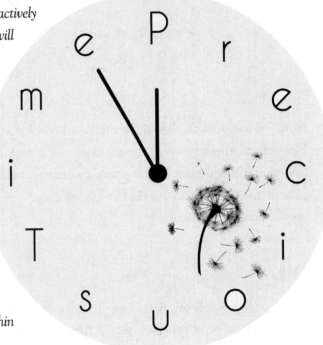

The term "Precious Time" was coined by my late husband, Bob Lehmberg, a palliative care physician who would tell patients and families, "You are now entering into Precious Time," to help them understand that death was nearing. We received handwritten notes from families of patients who had died, thanking Bob for letting them know they were within their window of Precious Time.

What might your Precious Time look and sound like? Would you use that term or call it something else? Whatever the name, this is the period to slow down and lean in. It might begin while a dying person is still communicative and then continue through active dying to the last exhale and even beyond, as there is no need to immediately rush or act. For some, caring for a deceased person's body might also be included in Precious Time, particularly if it's their belief that communication and connection is still possible and important.

Your objective is to interpret these nuances for yourself and then to make your deathbed wishes known to others.

CHAPTER 12

Contemplative Planning for the End of Life

Now, you will work through the components of the deathbed space to help clarify your personalized plan. Please note, the following template does not constitute a medical or legal form, yet its contents can inform and complement advance care documents. Make sure to check out the appendices for additional planning tools. For now, answer the following questions to the degree that suits you and your needs. As always, peruse and choose.

Who?

Who are the people of your *village*? Your inner circle? Your family—biological or chosen? And do you have a go-to or point person, steady in their reliability, whom you can trust and lean on?

_____

_____

_____

_____

Not everyone has close friends or family members, although there are often kind-hearted, generous people around who are eager to step in when asked. Think about your neighborhood, people you have helped previously, as well as any groups you belong to or have been a part of in the past, such as faith communities, book clubs, sports or activity teams, volunteer or parenting groups, and so forth. Branch out and try not to discount people's willingness before checking with them first.

Next, brainstorm an encompassing list of all the important tasks you complete yourself—daily, weekly, monthly, seasonally, and annually—that you would need assistance with during your final days and after your death. Include practical ones as well as any that hold personal significance.

Tasks	Helpers
_____	_____
_____	_____
_____	_____
_____	_____
_____	_____
_____	_____
_____	_____
_____	_____

Now, mark with a star the items on your list that are absolutely necessary—as in, if they didn't get done, there would be a disastrous, dangerous, or harmful outcome. This will help you prioritize. You can go a step further and rank the items with a certain number of stars, such as, three stars for necessary, two stars for important, and one star for preferable.

Return to your list of tasks and begin filling in names of any potential helpers next to each one, focusing on the necessary items first. Identify who might be willing and adept. Whom would you trust? Whom could you count on? If you don't have a robust natural network, you can mark down titles of roles you might need to include—paid or volunteer—such as "dog walker" or "estate planner."

Are there gaps in your list? Are there extraneous tasks that you might be able to cross out upon honest reflection? Is there anything you could work toward completing or arranging now to alleviate some of the burden in the future?

_____

_____

_____

_____

This exercise not only reveals your to-do list, but it also speaks to your roles and sense of identity. Letting go of responsibilities can be an impossibly challenging aspect of declining health and the anticipatory grief that often accompanies death planning. Letting go isn't easy. Pause to process this and consider journaling and self-nurturance practices, if desired.

_____

_____

_____

_____

Deathbed Gathering

In addition to recognizing what life tasks you might need assistance with and who might fill those roles, you also need to think about who might be at the bedside while you're at the end of life. Some of us know who we'd want there; certain faces might immediately come to mind. Or this might not be so clear initially. You might find yourself returning to this segment to make edits and add details as we continue to explore the other aspects of end-of-life planning.

To start, think about your core circle of trusted companions and expand from there. Here's an example—which may or may not match your current constellation of connections—to encourage your brainstorm.

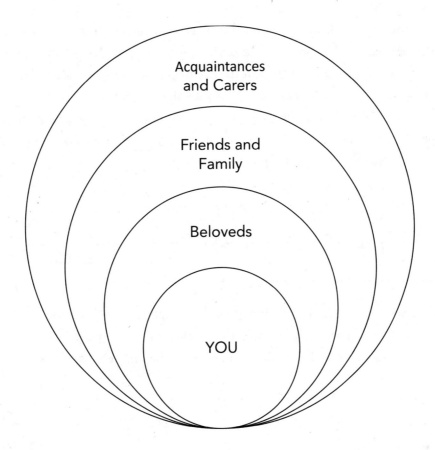

Think about these circles in regard to who you have available and how close you might want to draw them into your dying experience. To help you visualize the experience, consider the common phases of a natural dying process:

1. The time when someone ends curative treatments and focuses on comfort care

2. The duration when energy and attention start to decrease and a person requires more support

3. The period of increased sleepiness

4. The active dying process when a person can no longer interact much or at all with those present.

You might want certain visitors to come during specific phases and not others. You might also want periods of solitude along the way.

There's a spectrum of approaches to this part of planning:

Mine ➜ Ours ➜ Yours

Some people decide to draft their most ideal scenario and cling to that strategy very rigidly. That would be the "mine" version. The opposite end of the spectrum, "yours," would mean putting aside all your personal hopes to instead think only about the needs and preferences of others. You might find the middle ground, "ours," to be most realistic and healthy for all involved.

In this way, you'll lead with your wishes, yet take into consideration how well others will be able to actualize the plan. This can help everyone avoid disappointment, overwhelm, and regret. Take some time now to make some notes about your best approach.

_____

_____

_____

Now, arrange your preferred support team around you. Who are they? Factor in all your potential needs—physical, practical, emotional, psychological, social, medical, spiritual, holistic, and informational—as you create your care circle. List people in terms of their names or roles.

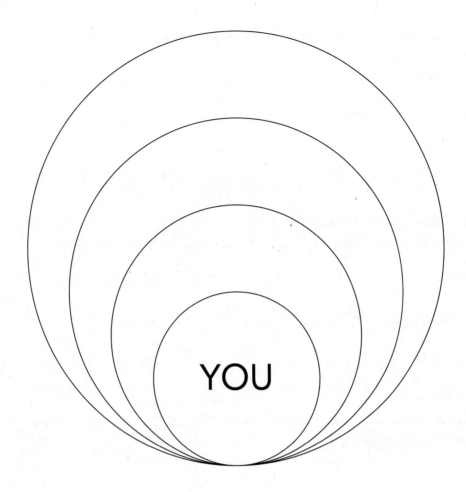

You can download a copy of this image at http://www.newharbinger.com/51369.

What attributes do these chosen people have that you appreciate? What connections do you share? What offerings could they supply?

_____

_____

_____

_____

_____

Who, if anyone, would you prefer *not* to be present (at all or during certain times)?

_____

_____

Reflections

How was that to surround yourself with the presence of your selected circle? Can you identify any potential gaps in coverage? If so, how might you address them?

_____

_____

_____

If there are certain people you don't want to visit your deathbed, it can bring up strong emotions and memories. Take care to lean on supports, such as a compassionate listener as well as coping techniques.

Please keep in mind that not everyone will be able to pause their own life to become part of this journey with you. Also, not everyone will feel emotionally capable to do so even if circumstances are agreeable. Refusals can seem like a personal affront. *Am I not important enough? Do I not mean anything to this person after all?* Keep in mind that resistance to being involved in another person's deathbed planning stems more often from fear than disregard.

You might want to have conversations now (or soon) to gauge people's willingness and to explain your wishes. You might even make a pact with certain loved ones to support one another during challenging times, including dying and grieving. Reciprocity can be a helpful way to respond to the anxiety death planning can provoke; the two of you can find reassurance in each other's vow of support.

What?

Now that you have envisioned who might be by your side, let's think about what might transpire during your final phase. In what ways can your community honor you? What special ceremonies or personal touches would you like to include in your end-of-life experience? Consider any religious or spiritual practices as well as:

Readings: favorite books, poetry, mantras, religious or spiritual texts, messages from loved ones, and so forth

_____

_____

_____

Visualizations or relaxations: prerecorded or written scripts (include what they're called and where they're located)

_____

_____

_____

Rituals: fully planned or basic wishes (include what they're called and where they're located)

_____

_____

_____

Scents: floral, mild essential oils, candles, incense, favorite foods baking or cooking

_____

_____

_____

An altar with sacred objects: focal points like postcards and photos, healing stones, figurines

_____

_____

_____

Lighting: fake or real candles, dim or bright overheads

_____

_____

_____

You might rank your ideas according to their importance. What is an absolute priority? What would be nice but not necessary? Mark items on your list with stars or numbers to illustrate their rank.

Now consider some additional *what* questions.

What would you like to be wearing? What material of sheets and blankets would you prefer?

_____

_____

What aspects of your appearance are important to you in terms of grooming (shaving, hair style, makeup, and so forth)?

_____

_____

Another aspect of your "what" is sound. It is believed that hearing is the very last sense to fade. Of course, there's a notable difference between hearing and paying attention. Yet even if our focus or consciousness might be concentrated elsewhere during active dying (such as a life review or spiritual experience, perhaps), it seems wise to assume we might, in fact, be listening and to plan for it—just in case.

What sounds do you imagine wanting to hear during your final weeks? Days? Minutes? Would you enjoy hearing people read to you or share memories? How about white noise, sounds from nature, or music?

_____

_____

_____

_____

Returning once more to my Aunt Nancy's impactful death, I had suggested to one of my cousins that they play her favorite tunes. Not only did the music muffle the hospital buzzes and beeps, it also created a personalized atmosphere. When she took her final breath and cried that single tear, the Beach Boys were softly serenading her.

Some music thanatologists and threshold singers believe songs can soothe us during the time leading up to the vigil period, yet they theorize that familiar music might anchor us to our body when death is imminent, thus interrupting the process. For that reason, they suggest playing or singing unfamiliar songs during the final hours. You might ponder how this theory lands with you. Does it resonate?

If it appeals, make your own playlist for the end of life in the following exercise. This list says a lot about you. It reflects your taste in music, and it offers a stroll down memory lane if you choose to include songs from various eras.

My deathbed playlist

Music to:

Soothe

_____

_____

_____

_____

_____

_____

Uplift

_____

_____

_____

_____

_____

_____

Reminisce

_____

_____

_____

_____

_____

_____

_____

Reflections

How was that to make your personal playlist? Did you decide to listen to any songs while building your set?

_____

_____

Music can transport us—mentally and emotionally. It can bring us back to our past or send us some place in our imagination. It can shift our mood.

You might be inclined to take this exercise a step further and actually create some playlists for yourself. Title each appropriately so your care circle knows when and how to use them. You might build a specific set for vigil and then have some other lists prepared to either bolster your mood or calm your nerves, depending on the situation.

If you don't have the means or expertise to pull together songs into a usable form, look to your care circle. People often appreciate the opportunity to offer help, especially in specific ways.

When?

We are intentionally skipping any *when* exercises. Within the end-of-life realm, there is mystery. When a person is terminally ill, medical care providers can sometimes provide an estimate of time remaining, generally in the range of "years to months," "months to weeks," "weeks to days," or "days to hours." A prognosis is a best-guess prediction made up of statistical averages blended with individual health factors. And there are always outliers and exceptions, making the *when* far more difficult to pin down.

If knowing *when* becomes a pressing issue during your journey, you might expand your focus to include a conversation with care providers about what to expect. Ask about commonalities, signs, and stages regarding the last phase of life as well as supportive strategies to relieve any suffering that might arise.

Where?

Some people have a certain place in mind for their time of dying. They might have a very strong preference for being in a particular room for their last breath. Some people want to be "home" (wherever that may be) or at the home of a friend or family member. Some people hope to be in a hospice house, receiving medical care within a homelike environment. Others feel safest in a hospital, due to familiarity, past health episodes, or current complications. You might have a location picked out for yourself already, or this might be a new line of thinking you haven't yet pondered.

Often, what's more important than a specific address is how the space itself feels. What's more, we cannot always predict in advance where someone will receive the level of care that will be needed. Sometimes, due to challenging symptoms or unrelenting suffering, people have to change plans unexpectedly. This can seem like yet another loss. When we acknowledge this possibility ahead of time though, we can discuss contingency plans and environmental features that might be adaptable to wherever the dying experience ends up happening.

Keep these considerations in mind as you work through the following visualization and prompts while refining your priorities and wishes.

Visualization Exercise: Your Where

Set aside five to ten minutes to visualize yourself on your deathbed, whenever the experience of dying might happen in the future. You can choose to actually lie down and close your eyes for this exercise, if that's appealing. You might want to listen to your vigil playlist quietly. Immerse yourself fully in the experience, focusing on finding deep comfort in and around yourself. When you've reached a comfortable level of relaxation and clarity in your visualization, take a few moments to look around for details (in your imagination).

Where is this place for you? How does it feel? How does it smell? Are there aromas in the air? What is around you? How is it set up? Are there sounds? Who is present, if anyone? What are you wearing? Are there special items surrounding you?

When you're ready, bring yourself back to the current moment and write down everything you noticed during your visualization. Now, describe your ideal deathbed location in detail. Also, note what it is about this place that feels inviting and comforting.

_____

_____

_____

_____

_____

_____

_____

_____

_____

Given that sometimes people must move to a different location based on care needs, what alternative places would be acceptable to you? What aspects of your ideal location could be replicated elsewhere?

_____

_____

_____

What is most essential about your *where*?

_____

_____

_____

Why?

While there is no need to feel pressured to defend your choices, it can be useful for others to learn more about your reasoning. Why are your stated preferences important to you? Why do you feel the way you do?

_____

_____

_____

_____

_____

To help further convey your *why*, contemplate your values and priorities—your guideposts in life. Feel free to revisit your beliefs list in chapter 10 for inspiration.

Share your most strongly held beliefs, hopes, morals, and ideals:

_____

_____

_____

_____

_____

_____

_____

_____

_____

Define what "courage" means to you and share a story that illustrates courage:

_____

_____

_____

_____

_____

_____

_____

_____

Describe your very best day from start to finish:

_____

_____

_____

_____

_____

How might you infuse some of your stated guideposts, thoughts on courage, or parts of your best day into your end-of-life planning?

_____

_____

_____

_____

_____

How?

In terms of "how," we're not going to delve too deeply into exactly how you might die as it's a complicated, largely abstract topic. Most of us will not have a true say in how our life actually ends, in terms of the cause and timing. Some people imagine they'd like to fall asleep and never wake up. Others think they'd like to be lucid, perhaps surrounded by loved ones or the sounds of prayers or chants. One aspect of your *how* you can consider is your preferred degree of alertness as you near death.

You can keep these factors in mind:

- Patients can talk through different pain medications with medical care providers to understand potential risks, benefits, and side effects, and to discuss any worries about overuse or dependence. Pain medication can significantly reduce suffering (when present).

- Additionally, there are other comfort measures to consider, like position changes, attentive personal care, and integrative healing modalities (for example therapeutic touch and massage, energy healing, acupuncture, animal-assisted therapy, aromatherapy, dietary support, music therapy, meditation, and many others). Again, these are conversations people can have with care providers throughout a serious or terminal illness.

At this juncture, whatever your current health status, you might ask yourself: *During my time of dying, would I rather be heavily sedated and completely comfortable or alert even if I'm enduring some pain? Or somewhere in between?*

Jot down your initial thoughts and any questions you might direct to your care providers.

_____

_____

_____

_____

_____

Deathbed Invitations

One factor of your *how* is how you might welcome visitors into your dying space. A person's dying journey is a particularly intimidating period. Often, people feel nervous to show up and be present during times of intensity. *What will I say? What should I do?* Worries can keep some people away completely. Consequently, dying can become very lonely.

A doula once shared a heart-rending story about supporting her friend through the end of life. Her friend wanted to spend more time with those he knew and cared about. He noticed that as he became more sick, fewer people stopped by or scheduled visits. Recognizing nervousness as the main issue, he asked the doula to send out a message to his community. "Come and say the wrong thing," he implored. He wanted people to be close by and to come freely, without being afraid of him or the situation.

If you think you would appreciate and enjoy visitors while on your deathbed, think about how you might encourage them to come spend time with you. What message might you send out? How could it best reflect your voice, personality, and hopes? It might be one line or a paragraph. You might remind your village that you are still you ("I am not my illness. I'm me.") and that you'd like to remain connected.

_____

_____

_____

_____

_____

_____

In addition to that message, you can also create a welcome note for people to read as they enter your dying space. This can provide a frame of reference and some ideas for your time together. For example:

Welcome! I'm so pleased you've come to visit. My hope for our time is that you might leave your shoes, keys, devices, and worries behind so we can be together without distraction. If I'm awake, feel free to talk with me. I'd love to hear about your life these days and maybe stories of the times we've shared together. If I'm asleep, feel free to read aloud from any of the books I have on the side table or to just sit quietly. Before you leave, please add a written message to me (memories or wishes) in my visitor book so I can cherish our relationship even after you leave.

Thinking about what brings you comfort and the various wishes you've already identified in this chapter, how could you welcome visitors into your dying experience? Write out your personalized version of a welcome note.

_____

_____

_____

_____

_____

_____

_____

_____

_____

After-Death Options

Another *how* question is how you want your body cared for following your death. If you already have such requests articulated within your advance directives, this can be a chance to double-check that they're still accurate. If you are just beginning this type of planning, gently work through the following questions, going at your own pace as you feel comfortable.

Immediately following your death, what would you like your loved ones or carers to do or not do?

_____

_____

_____

Is there a certain amount of time you would like your body to be undisturbed?

_____

_____

Is there a certain amount of time within which you want your final disposition (how you're laid to rest) to occur?

_____

_____

Are there any rituals or ceremonies you want others to carry out (for example washing and anointing your body, dressing you in certain garb, or reciting certain prayers, rites, chants, or poetry) or any other cultural, spiritual, or religious practices you would like to request for after your final exhale?

_____

_____

_____

_____

Would you like to donate tissues or organs for transplantation, if possible? Or gift your physical vessel as a whole body donation to medical science?

_____

_____

Are you planning to have a wake or "viewing"? If so, would this happen at home? (Note: Your friends and family members would need to make legal and practical arrangements, perhaps with guidance from a funeral director, home funeral guide, or death doula.) Or are you planning to have a wake in a funeral home in advance or in place of services? Or would you prefer no wake at all?

_____

_____

What are you planning for your final disposition?

Here are some options to consider (mainly sourced from the United States):

Cremation

- Fire cremation (in some places, open-air cremation on a funeral pyre is also an option)
- Water cremation, called alkaline hydrolysis, or "aquamation"—a more eco-friendly alternative to fire cremation that uses water, alkali, and heat

Burial

- Green or natural burial (bypassing embalming and concrete vaults while opting for biodegradable materials, like raw wooden or cardboard caskets or simple shrouds)
- Conservation burial, namely, natural burial on lands protected by a recognized conservation land trust entity
- Home burial
- Contemporary cemetery burial (in-ground, mausoleum or crypt, burial alone or alongside loved ones, veterans' cemetery)
- Burial at sea

Natural organic reduction, also called human composting, available in an increasing number of locations

Spend some time researching what is legal and available to you, and then consider what is affordable and personally appealing.

Finally, depending on your preferences, decide if you would want a gravesite of some sort. Will people be able to visit a physical place to mourn and remember you (like a cemetery or memorial garden) or simply access your essence within their memories and hearts?

_____

_____

_____

_____

_____

In places outside of the United States and throughout history, there is and has been an endless variety of after-death traditions. You might take time to research and explore them to expand your awareness. We don't know what we don't know until we learn about it. It's eye-opening to acknowledge that for as long as humans have lived, we've died. Reflect on the practices of your ancestors and also research to see what else is possible in your area. End-of-life choices can be a reflection of the kind of person you are and what has been important to you. What might honor you best?

Celebration of Life

Our next *how* topic is how you want your life to be commemorated. In this activity, you will be planning your own celebration of life. Organizing your own end-of-life event doesn't mean you (or others) need to follow through on the plan necessarily. Some people will find meaning in working through the details simply for the sake of contemplation. (You can download this activity from http://www.newharbinger.com/51369.)

Planning. Your celebration of life could be a pre-funeral (also known as a "living funeral") to be held while you're still alive or a memorial service after your death. Both have similar elements you can include. When planning your event, once again utilize the *who, what, where, when, why,* and *how* questions to round out specifics.

Who would you like to be present? Are you envisioning a big affair or quiet gathering? In-person guests or online? A hybrid? One of each?

_____

_____

_____

_____

_____

What would you like to have happen during the event? Readings? Planned eulogies or speeches? Open invitations to speak? Music? Rituals? Religious or spiritual prayers or practices? Food and drinks (catered, potluck, or supplied by close friends and family)? Framed photos? Collages? Slide shows? A visitor book for messages? Parting gifts for attendees (customized candles, seeds for planting, bestowal offerings, and so forth)?

_____

_____

_____

_____

_____

When might the event happen? Unlike your general end-of-life planning in this chapter where we bypassed activities regarding the timing, you might have more say about when a celebration of life happens. If you're intending to hold a living funeral, then sometimes a timeline does accelerate due to a decline in health, but you might have a preferred day of the week, month, or season in mind. When planning an after-death service, you might want it to occur a certain number of days after your passing, or on a preferred day of the week, or on a specific date.

_____

_____

_____

_____

_____

Where might the event occur? First calculate your budget. How much have you reserved for this expense, and how much will others potentially contribute? Then, think about the location. Indoors or outside? A backyard, place of worship, burial site, or a less obvious space that could accommodate such a request, like a library, restaurant, armory, retreat center, museum, golf course, park, beach, school or university, or another meaningful-to-you location. What venue would work well for you, your guests, and your activities? What other locations might be acceptable alternative locations in case your first choice isn't available?

_____

_____

_____

_____

_____

_____

Why hold a celebration of life? The connections we make and the impact we have while alive matter. And they're worth honoring. Even if yours has been a quiet existence, you likely have accomplishments to commemorate. Undoubtedly, you have overcome obstacles and hardship. You have had relationships with others. Plus, a celebration of life is an invaluable opportunity to communally grieve and reminisce. It can facilitate the healthy integration of a loss. With these explanations in mind, why hold yours? What hopes do you have for it?

_____

_____

_____

_____

_____

How will this plan come together? How much can you arrange ahead of time? How much assistance do you need now, and how much help will be needed for the actual event?

_____

_____

_____

_____

_____

Living on in Memories

In this final *how* activity, we'll focus on how you'd like to be remembered. First, contemplate these opening questions: *How do you hope others will remember you? How do you think they will actually remember you? How might others describe your personality? How might you live on in the memories of others?*

_____

_____

_____

_____

_____

_____

You can use your responses above to now write your own obituary. While an obituary is a way to inform others of a death, it can also be a means to succinctly recount a life. Not everyone ends up having a published death notice. Some people state their preference for or against this ritual while alive; for others, their next of kin decides on their behalf. Regardless of outcome, it can be an enlightening exercise to write your own. It might never be shared, it could be published verbatim, or it might be a draft your loved ones use to complete the final version.

Before penning it, think about your style and what tone would be best. *How would you want your obituary to read or come across to others? What effect do you hope it might have? Do you prefer a traditional format, or would you rather give it some flair, humor, or poignancy? Do you want to keep it strictly "positive," as in the good times only?* Here are some opening prompts to start brainstorming. You can utilize much of your writing from previous activities in this section.

Biography (timeline and relationships)

_____

_____

_____

_____

_____

_____

_____

_____

_____

_____

_____

_____

Meaningful moments

_____

_____

_____

_____

_____

Accomplishments and sources of pride

_____

_____

_____

_____

_____

Personality traits

_____

_____

_____

_____

Hobbies and interests

_____

_____

_____

_____

Personal mantra (words you live by or epitaph, an inscription on a tombstone)

_____

_____

_____

Encouraging advice about life and how to best honor you

_____

_____

_____

Now that you have come up with the potential components of an obituary, you might want to write an organized, more polished version. Feel free to follow a traditional template or break the mold.

My obituary

_____

_____

_____

_____

_____

_____

_____

Whether you have chosen to complete just a few of the previous end-of-life planning activities or all of them, you have done an immense amount of internal work requiring enormous energy. Take a deep, cleansing breath. Praise yourself for these efforts and reward yourself with a truly nourishing act of self-love.

Part VII

Parting Gifts: Saying Goodbye

Much of the work we've done throughout the book resides within the theoretical realm. You have been imagining what your own end-of-life journey might entail while practicing self-compassion, processing any anxieties, and looking back on previous experiences. This work is undeniably valuable. We can also expand our understanding by learning directly from people facing death.

So, what do people who are dying talk about most often? What do they generally care about in the end?

As a deathcare provider, I have witnessed some notable commonalities. When people with terminal illnesses near their final moments, material goods and money tend not to matter as much. As their world gets smaller—going from days spent out in the community, to staying within the bounds of home, to remaining within the confines of one bed or chair—their focus often narrows. People turn inward, contemplating their legacy or impact as well as relationships.

In her book *Dear Death*, Diane Button (2021, 141) pulls from her experience as a death doula and writes, "At the end of life…we will care about people and animals. We will want to know that we offered kindness to a hurting planet and to those in need. We will care about loving and being loved. We will care about leaving the world a little bit better than we found it."

Similarly, hospice chaplain and author Kerry Egan (2017) finds those she serves often speak about the love they felt and gave in addition to love they didn't receive or know how to offer. Egan goes on to explain that people don't live their lives through theology and theories. Instead, we live real life within our family units—the biological families we're born into and those we form, including with close friends. This is where we create our lives; this is where we find meaning; and this is where our purpose becomes clear.

What if we could access this narrowed focus and clarity before death calls? What if we could live *now* in all the ways we might wish we had when our time is very short? Might we avoid some regret? Mend some relationships? Heal some hurts? Reprioritize our days to honor what we hold dear?

If you are currently in good or stable health, imagine you just received a prognosis of a year to live, or a month, or just a week. If you are currently ill, honestly and gently assess your energy and concerns. Now ask yourself: *What matters are seeking my attention right now? What has been delayed or forgotten that I might act upon while there's still time?*

_____

_____

_____

_____

_____

_____

CHAPTER 13

The Final Farewell

You've made it to the last few prompts of the workbook—congratulations!

Interpret and answer them however you like with either inspirational, light-hearted, or instructional words. You might freewrite in complete sentences or draft lists. You might also include poems, quotes, or song lyrics. Whether you direct these words to a specific person or people, yourself, or humanity at large, tap into your inner wisdom and voice.

This is your book; these are your reflections.

Words to grieve by...

_____

_____

_____

_____

_____

_____

_____

My wish for you is...

_____

_____

_____

_____

_____

_____

_____

_____

Now, we must embody the principles we have reviewed. The importance of acknowledging impermanence and practicing the art of goodbye cannot be overlooked. You have reached the end of your mortality awareness journey within this workbook—a rite of passage in and of itself.

As part of this experience, you have likely deconstructed some old ways of thinking as you made space for new possibilities and perspectives. You delved into the unknown—the liminal space—opening yourself up to the discomfort and liberation found in healing and growth. And now, you reemerge, incorporating all you've learned.

So, how has this death wellness undertaking been for you, dear reader? Surprising? Enlightening? Frustrating? Emotional?

Whatever it has entailed, may it propel you onward, deeper into your quest. May this moment present as a gratifying culmination. May it be an invitation to pause, look back at all you have discovered, and then gaze ahead at all that awaits. As long as you're breathing, you will be navigating the mess and brilliance of being human—of being mortal.

What remains?

Values Worksheet for Advance Care Planning

Below are some questions to consider as you make decisions about your health care preferences. They come from the Values and Priorities Worksheet in the Compassion and Choices End of Life Decision Guide (available for free at https://compassionandchoices.org/resource/eoldgt). You may want to write down your answers and provide copies to your family members and health care providers, or simply use the questions as "food for thought" and a basis for discussion.

How important to you are the following items?

	Very important				Not important
Letting nature take its course	4	3	2	1	0
Preserving quality of life	4	3	2	1	0
Staying true to my spiritual beliefs and traditions	4	3	2	1	0
Living as long as possible, regardless of quality of life	4	3	2	1	0
Being independent	4	3	2	1	0
Being comfortable and as pain-free as possible	4	3	2	1	0
Leaving good memories for my family and friends	4	3	2	1	0
Making a contribution to medical research or teaching	4	3	2	1	0
Being able to relate to family and friends	4	3	2	1	0
Being free of physical limitations	4	3	2	1	0
Being mentally alert and competent	4	3	2	1	0
Being able to leave money to family, friends, or charity	4	3	2	1	0
Dying more quickly rather than lingering	4	3	2	1	0
Avoiding expensive care	4	3	2	1	0

What will be important to you when you are dying (for example physical comfort, no pain, family members present)?

_____

_____

_____

_____

From the Compassion and Choices End of Life Decision Guide (Compassion and Choices 2022).

How do you feel about the use of the life-sustaining measures in the following situations?

- Terminal illness

- Permanent coma

- Irreversible chronic illness

- Dementia

_____

_____

_____

_____

Do you have strong feelings about particular medical procedures?

- Mechanical breathing (respirator)

- Cardiopulmonary resuscitation (CPR)

- Artificial nutrition and hydration

- Hospital intensive care

- Pain-relief medication

- Antibiotics

- Chemo or radiation therapy

- Surgery

_____

_____

_____

_____

From the Compassion and Choices End of Life Decision Guide (Compassion and Choices 2022).

What limitations to your physical or mental health would affect the health care decisions you would make?

_____

_____

_____

_____

Would you want to be placed in a nursing home or care facility if your condition warranted?

_____

_____

Would you prefer hospice care, with the goal of keeping you comfortable in your home during the final period of your life, as an alternative to hospitalization?

_____

_____

In general, do you wish to participate or share in making decisions about your health care and treatment?

_____

_____

_____

From the Compassion and Choices End of Life Decision Guide (Compassion and Choices 2022).

Would you always want to know the truth about your condition, treatment options, and the chance of success of treatments?

_____

_____

_____

Advance Directive

Once you're comfortable stating your values and priorities, you're ready to complete your advance directive. It clarifies your end-of-life preferences if you become unable to make or communicate medical treatment decisions yourself. Typically, the advance directive includes a living will ("what I want") and a medical durable power of attorney ("who will speak for me"). It may also include other documents.

If you're within the United States, you can locate your state's forms on the Compassion and Choices website: https://compassionandchoices.org/in-your-state.

Physician Orders for Life Sustaining Treatment (POLST)

POLSTs are specific treatment orders that can be written by a physician. To learn more about them, start with our online DNR/POLST resource (http://www.compassionandchoices.org/end-of-life-planning). You can also visit the national POLST website to learn more and see your state's form (http://www.polst.org/programs-in-your-state). If you feel you need a POLST, you must complete the form with your physician.

From the Compassion and Choices End of Life Decision Guide (Compassion and Choices 2022).

"Organized for the End" Task List

Review the following list to help determine what specific information will be useful for your loved ones or care partners at the end of your life—or during a medical emergency. You might choose to add your details here within this section. If you do, feel free to cross out items that don't apply and add other things that aren't listed. As an alternative, you can utilize a journal for your list or write it out on a separate sheet of paper. Just make sure to keep this document in a safe, private spot that's accessible for your loved ones or care partners. You might also make a copy of it to share with a trusted person for safekeeping. (You can download this activity from http://www.newharbinger.com/51369.)

Personal Information: address, phone, medical conditions and medications, health insurance policies

_____

_____

_____

_____

_____

_____

_____

_____

Contact List:

Personal: family, friends, neighbors, coworkers

_____

_____

_____

_____

_____

Professional: lawyer, accountant, insurance agent, tax professional

_____

_____

_____

_____

_____

Health-care providers

_____

_____

_____

_____

_____

Location of Important Documents

Birth, marriage, divorce, agreements, settlements

_____

_____

_____

Social security card, license or other identification card, citizenship, armed forces discharge papers

_____

_____

_____

Vehicles, household bills and utilities, insurance policies, titles, deeds

_____

_____

_____

Tax returns, social security and disability payments, investments, retirement, pension plans

_____

_____

_____

Business files (if an owner or self-employed)

_____

_____

_____

Advance care planning, living will, healthcare proxy, DNR, trusts, power of attorney

_____

_____

_____

Pre-death planning: arrangements, payments, obituary, wishes for services

_____

_____

_____

_____

Remembrance gifts (digital and physical)

_____

_____

_____

Financial Information

Bank accounts, debit and credit cards, mortgages, loans, safe deposit box and keys, cash stashes

_____

_____

_____

_____

Logins and Passwords

Email, online business accounts, social media

_____

_____

_____

_____

Pets

Instructions and wishes

_____

_____

_____

Location of Personal Items

_____

_____

_____

Additional Instructions

_____

_____

_____

_____

_____

_____

_____

_____

_____

Thank You

There are so many amazing people who were part of this journey—my ancestors, friends, family members, clients, colleagues, and those in my doula community certainly stand out. No act of encouragement has gone unnoticed or unappreciated!

Thank you, Ryan Buresh, for the invitation to author this book. It was clearly bouncing around in my mind, and this experience has proven an incredibly gratifying. My thanks to Vicraj Gill for helping to organize my initially unwieldy musings. I didn't anticipate using the word *ultimately* so many times, but I'm happy to see it scattered throughout the chapters. And my appreciation to Gretel Hakanson for your keen eye and encouraging feedback. I really enjoyed working with the entire team at New Harbinger!

Special thanks to the people who read drafts (or parts of them), including Roberta MacDonald, Kim Callinan, Heather Caulfield, Charley MacMartin, Diane Button, Gretchen Ward, and Jackie Weinstock. Your suggestions were invaluable, as was your support! An additional nod to Diane Button for the invitation to visit your slice of paradise. I'm not sure I could have finished the manuscript without that writing retreat.

For more notes on gratitude, you'll have to visit page 22 of my death journal…

Resources

Caring Info (Resources) https://www.caringinfo.org/

Compassion and Choices (Planning) https://www.compassionandchoices.org/

Conservation Burial Alliance https://www.conservationburialalliance.org/definitions.html

Death Café https://deathcafe.com/

End of Life University Podcast https://www.eoluniversity.com/podcast

Five Wishes (Advance Directives) https://www.fivewishes.org/

Funeral Consumers Alliance https://funerals.org/

Green Burial Council https://www.greenburialcouncil.org/

International Association for Indigenous Aging https://iasquared.org/

National Asian Pacific Center on Aging https://www.napca.org/

National End-of-Life Doula Alliance https://www.nedalliance.org/

National Caucus and Center on Black Aging https://ncba-aging.org/

National Council on Aging https://ncoa.org/

National Hispanic Council on Aging https://nhcoa.org/

National Home Funeral Alliance https://www.homefuneralalliance.org/

The National Indian Council on Aging https://www.nicoa.org/

SAGE (Advocacy and Services for LGBTQ+ Elders) https://www.sageusa.org/

References

Arnoldy, F. L. 2018. *Cultivating the Doula Heart: Essentials of Compassionate Care*. Hinesburg, VT: Contemplative Doula.

Banks, A. 2010. "Humans Are Hardwired for Connection? Neurobiology 101 for Parents, Educators, Practitioners, and the General Public." Interview by *Wellesley Centers for Women*. Wellesley Centers for Women, Wellesley College, September 15, 2010. https://www.wcwonline.org/2010/humans-are -hardwired-for-connection-neurobiology-101-for-parents-educators-practitioners-and-the-general -public.

Becker, E. 1973. *The Denial of Death*. New York: Free Press.

Bronfenbrenner, U. 1979. *The Ecology of Human Development: Experiments by Nature and Design*. Cambridge, MA: Harvard University Press.

Button, D. 2021. *Dear Death*. Waialua, HI: Better World Publishing.

Chödrön, P. 2000. *When Things Fall Apart: Heart Advice for Difficult Times*. Boulder, CO: Shambhala Publications.

Chödrön, P. 2003. *Comfortable with Uncertainty: 108 Teachings on Cultivating Fearlessness and Compassion*. Boulder, CO: Shambhala Publications.

Compassion and Choices. 2022. "My End-of-Life Decisions: An Advance Planning Guide and Toolkit." *Compassion & Choices*. https://www.compassionandchoices.org/resources/eoldgt.

Covey, S. 2004. *The Seven Habits of Highly Effective People*. New York: Simon and Schuster.

Dor-Ziderman, Y., A. Lutz, and A. Goldstein. 2019. "Prediction-Based Neural Mechanisms for Shielding the Self from Existential Threat." *NeuroImage* 202:116080.

Ducharme, J. 2020. "COVID-19 Is Making America's Loneliness Epidemic Worse." *Time*, May 8, 2020. https://time.com/5833681/loneliness-covid-19/.

Egan, K. 2017. "What People Talk About Before Dying." *CNN Health*, December 20, 2017. https://www.cnn.com/2016/12/20/health/what-people-talk-about-before-dying-kerry-egan/index.html.

Elder, G. H., Jr., and M. J. Shanahan. 2006. "The Life Course and Human Development." In *Handbook of Child Psychology: Theoretical Models of Human Development*, edited by M. Lerner and W. Damon, 665–715. New York: John Wiley & Sons.

Erikson, E. H. 1950. *Childhood and Society*. New York: W. W. Norton & Company.

Ernest Becker Foundation. n.d. "Terror Management Theory." https://ernestbecker.org/resources/terror-management-theory/.

Firestone, L. 2013. "How to Identify Your Critical Inner Voice." *Psychology Today*, January 23, 2013. https://www.psychologytoday.com/us/blog/compassion-matters/201301/how-identify-your-critical-inner-voice.

Gibran, K. 1923. *The Prophet*. New York: Knopf.

Greenberg, J., T. Pyszczynski, and S. Solomon. 1986. "The Causes and Consequences of a Need for Self-Esteem: A Terror Management Theory." In *Public Self and Private Self*, edited by R. F. Baumeister, 189–212. New York: Springer-Verlag.

Gruman, J. 2021. "The Power of Rituals." *Psychology Today*, April 11, 2021. https://www.psychologytoday.com/us/blog/dont-forget-the-basil/202104/the-power-rituals.

Hamby. S. 2013. "Resilience and 4 Benefits of Sharing Your Story." *Psychology Today*, September 3, 2013. https://www.psychologytoday.com/us/blog/the-web-violence/201309/resilience-and-4-benefits-sharing-your-story.

Jimenez, G. E. 2002. "My Own Self-Care." *The Hospice Heart* (blog), July 16, 2022. https://www.thehospiceheart.net/post/my-own-self-care.

Juhl, J., and C. Routledge. 2015. "Putting the Terror in Terror Management Theory: Evidence That the Awareness of Death Does Cause Anxiety and Undermine Psychological Well-Being." *Current Directions in Psychological Science* 25: 99–103

Kumar, S. K. M. 2013. *Mindfulness for Prolonged Grief: A Guide to Healing after Loss When Depression, Anxiety, and Anger Won't Go Away.* Oakland, CA: New Harbinger Publications.

Lamas, T., J. J. Froh, R. A. Emmons, A. Mishra, and G. Bono. 2014. "Gratitude Interventions: A Review and Future Agenda." In *The Wiley Blackwell Handbook of Positive Psychological Interventions*, edited by A. C. Parks and S. M. Schueller, 3–19. London, UK: Wiley-Blackwell.

Niles, A. N., K. E. Haltom, C. M. Mulvenna, M. D. Lieberman, and A. L. Stanton. 2014. "Randomized Controlled Trial of Expressive Writing for Psychological and Physical Health: The Moderating Role of Emotional Expressivity." *Anxiety Stress Coping* 27: 1–17.

Norelli, S. K., A. Long, and J. M. Krepps. 2021. "Relaxation Techniques." In *StatPearls*. Treasure Island, FL: StatPearls Publishing.

Palmer, P. 2016. "The Gift of Presence, the Perils of Advice." *On Being* (blog), April 27, 2016. https://onbeing.org/blog/the-gift-of-presence-the-perils-of-advice/.

Pawlowski, A. 2021. "3 Biggest Regrets People Have at the End of Life." *Today*, March 22, 2021. https://www.today.com/health/3-biggest-regrets-people-have-end-life-t212521.

Pennebaker, J. 2021. "Using Expressive Writing to Heal Trauma." *The Weekend University*. Youtube video, 51:59, https://youtu.be/CjErOxiXqio.

Pollock, A. 2016. "Why I Don't Use the Word Forgiveness in Trauma Therapy." *Good Therapy* (blog), January 20, 2016. https://www.goodtherapy.org/blog/why-i-dont-use-the-word-forgiveness-in-trauma-therapy-0120164.

The Order of the Good Death. n.d. "Death Positive Movement." *The Order of the Good Death.* https://www.orderofthegooddeath.com/death-positive-movement/.

Remen, R. N. 2001. *My Grandfather's Blessings: Stories of Strength, Refuge, and Belonging.* New York: Riverhead Books.

Rites of Passage. 2015. "Stages of a Rite of Passage." *Rites of Passage.* https://wildernessquest.org/stages-of-a-rite-of-passage/.

Ryan, R. M., and E. L. Deci. 2017. *Self-Determination Theory: Basic Psychological Needs in Motivation, Development, and Wellness.* New York: Guilford Press.

Ryan, R., and E. Deci. 2020. "Intrinsic and Extrinsic Motivation from a Self-Determination Theory Perspective: Definitions, Theory, Practices, and Future Directions." *Contemporary Educational Psychology* 61:101860.

Salzberg, S. 2015. "Compassion: A Way of Being in the World." *Sharon Salzberg* (blog), April 5, 2015. https://www.sharonsalzberg.com/compassion-a-way-of-being-in-the-world/.

Schenker, Y., M. A. Dew, C. F. Reynolds, R. M. Arnold, G. A. Tiver, and A. E. Barnato. 2015. "Development of a Post-Intensive Care Unit Storytelling Intervention for Surrogates Involved in Decisions to Limit Life-Sustaining Treatment." *Palliative & Supportive Care* 13: 451–463.

Sansone, R. A., and L. A. Sansone. 2010. "Gratitude and Well-Being." *Psychiatry* 7: 18–22.

Shelton, L. G. 2019. *The Bronfenbrenner Primer: A Guide to Develecology.* New York: Routledge.

Snape, D., and S. Manclossi. 2018. "Recommended National Indicators of Loneliness." *Office for National Statistics*, December 5, 2018. https://www.ons.gov.uk/peoplepopulationandcommunity /wellbeing/compendium/nationalmeasurementofloneliness/2018/recommendednational indicatorsofloneliness.

Tartakovsky, M. 2016. "Connecting to Your Core Self." *PsychCentral* (blog), October 14, 2016. https://psychcentral.com/blog/connecting-to-your-core-self#1.

Wood, A. M., J. J. Froh, and A. W. A. Geraghty. 2010. "Gratitude and Well-Being: A Review and Theoretical Integration." *Clinical Psychology Review* 30: 890–905.

Yalom, I. D. 2008. *Staring at the Sun: Overcoming the Terror of Death.* San Francisco, CA: Jossey-Bass.

Francesca Lynn Arnoldy is a community doula and death literacy advocate. She authored *Cultivating the Doula Heart*, and she is a researcher with the Vermont Conversation Lab. Francesca was the original course developer of the University of Vermont's End-of-Life Doula Professional Certificate Programs. She regularly presents on life-and-death topics with hopes of encouraging people to support one another through times of intensity.

MORE BOOKS from
NEW HARBINGER PUBLICATIONS

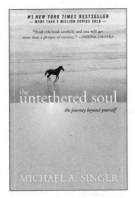
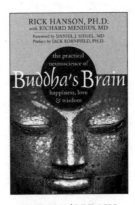
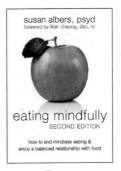
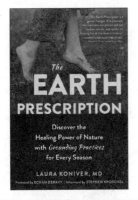
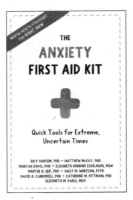
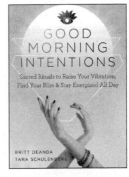

Did you know there are **free tools** you can download for this book?

Free tools are things like **worksheets, guided meditation exercises**, and **more** that will help you get the most out of your book.

You can download free tools for this book— whether you bought or borrowed it, in any format, from any source—from the New Harbinger website. All you need is a NewHarbinger.com account. Just use the URL provided in this book to view the free tools that are available for it. Then, click on the "download" button for the free tool you want, and follow the prompts that appear to log in to your NewHarbinger.com account and download the material.

You can also save the free tools for this book to your **Free Tools Library** so you can access them again anytime, just by logging in to your account! Just look for this button on the book's free tools page.

+ Save this to my free tools library

If you need help accessing or downloading free tools, visit **newharbinger.com/faq** or contact us at **customerservice@newharbinger.com**.